Dental Implants: An Evolving Discipline

Editor

ALEX M. GREENBERG

ORAL AND MAXILLOFACIAL SURGERY CLINICS OF NORTH AMERICA

www.oralmaxsurgery.theclinics.com

Consulting Editor
RICHARD H. HAUG

May 2015 • Volume 27 • Number 2

ELSEVIER

1600 John F. Kennedy Boulevard • Suite 1800 • Philadelphia, Pennsylvania, 19103-2899

http://www.oralmaxsurgery.theclinics.com

ORAL AND MAXILLOFACIAL SURGERY CLINICS OF NORTH AMERICA Volume 27, Number 2
May 2015 ISSN 1042-3699, ISBN-13: 978-0-323-37613-6

Editor: John Vassallo; j.vassallo@elsevier.com
Developmental Editor: Colleen Viola

Oral and Maxillofacial Surgery Clinics of North America (ISSN 1042-3699) is published quarterly by Elsevier Inc., 360 Park Avenue South, New York, NY 10010-1710. Months of issue are February, May, August, and November. Business and Editorial Offices: 1600 John F. Kennedy Blvd., Suite 1800, Philadelphia, PA 19103-2899. Periodicals postage paid at New York, NY and additional mailing offices. Subscription prices are $385.00 per year for US individuals, $567.00 per year for US institutions, $175.00 per year for US students and residents, $455.00 per year for Canadian individuals, $680.00 per year for Canadian institutions, $520.00 per year for international individuals, $680.00 per year for international institutions and $235.00 per year for Canadian and foreign students/residents. To receive student/resident rate, orders must be accompanied by name or affiliated institution, date of term, and the *signature* of program/residency coordinator on institution letterhead. Orders will be billed at individual rate until proof of status Is received. Foreign air speed delivery is included in all *Clinics* subscription prices. All prices are subject to change without notice. **POSTMASTER:** Send address changes to *Oral and Maxillofacial Surgery Clinics of North America,* Elsevier Periodicals Customer Service, 11830 Westline Industrial Drive, St. Louis, MO 63146. Tel: 1-800-654-2452 (U.S. and Canada); 314-447-8871 (outside U.S. and Canada). Fax: 314-447-8029. E-mail: journalscustomerservice-usa@elsevier.com (for print support); journalsonlinesupport-usa@elsevier.com (for online support).

Reprints. For copies of 100 or more, of articles in this publication, please contact the Commercial Reprints Department, Elsevier Inc., 360 Park Avenue South, New York, NY 10010-1710. Tel.: 212-633-3874; Fax: 212-633-3820; Email: reprints@elsevier.com.

Oral and Maxillofacial Surgery Clinics of North America is covered in *MEDLINE/PubMed (Index Medicus)*, *Science Citation Index Expanded (SciSearch®)*, *Journal Citation Reports/Science Edition*, and *Current Contents®/Clinical Medicine*.

Contributors

CONSULTING EDITOR

RICHARD H. HAUG, DDS
Professor and Chief, Oral Maxillofacial Surgery,
Carolinas Medical Center, Charlotte, North
Carolina

EDITOR

ALEX M. GREENBERG, DDS
Assistant Clinical Professor, Department of
Oral and Maxillofacial Surgery, Columbia
University College of Dental Medicine,
Attending, The New York Presbyterian
Hospital, The Mount Sinai Hospital, The Mount
Sinai Beth Israel Hospital, and The Mount Sinai
St. Luke's Roosevelt Hospital; Private Practice
Limited to Oral and Maxillofacial Surgery,
New York, New York

AUTHORS

TOMAS ALBREKTSSON, MD, PhD, RCPSG
Department of Prosthodontics, Faculty of
Odontology, Malmö University, Malmö,
Sweden; Department of Biomaterials,
Sahlgrenska Academy, Gothenburg
University, Gothenburg, Sweden

SHAHID R. AZIZ, DMD, MD, FACS
Professor, Department of Oral and
Maxillofacial Surgery, Rutgers School of
Dental Medicine, Newark, New Jersey

PIRIYA BOONSIRIPHANT, DDS
Postgraduate Resident, Advanced
Education Program in Prosthodontics,
Department of Prosthodontics, College of
Dentistry, New York University, New York,
New York

VINCENT CARRAO, DDS, MD, FACS
Chief and Program Director of Oral and
Maxillofacial Surgery, The Mount Sinai
Hospital, Mount Sinai Icahn School of
Medicine, New York, New York

ISABELLE DEMATTEIS, DDS
Chief Resident of Oral and Maxillofacial
Surgery, The Mount Sinai Hospital, Mount Sinai
Icahn School of Medicine, New York, New York

G. RAWLEIGH FISHER, DDS, MD
Private Practice, Lake Charles Oral and Facial
Surgery, Lake Charles, Louisiana

ERIC M. GENDEN, MD, FACS
Chairman and Professor, Department of
Otolaryngology/Head and Neck Surgery, The
Mount Sinai Hospital, New York, New York

ALEX M. GREENBERG, DDS
Assistant Clinical Professor, Department of
Oral and Maxillofacial Surgery, Columbia
University College of Dental Medicine,
Attending, The New York Presbyterian
Hospital, The Mount Sinai Hospital, The Mount
Sinai Beth Israel Hospital, and The Mount Sinai
St. Luke's Roosevelt Hospital; Private Practice
Limited to Oral and Maxillofacial Surgery,
New York, New York

CHRISTOPHER J. HAGGERTY, DDS, MD
Private Practice, Lakewood Oral and
Maxillofacial Surgery Specialists, Lee's
Summit, Missouri; Clinical Assistant
Professor, Oral and Maxillofacial Surgery,
University of Missouri-Kansas City, Kansas
City, Missouri

ALAN S. HERFORD, DDS, MD
Professor and Chair, Department of Oral and
Maxillofacial Surgery, Loma Linda University,
Loma Linda, California

JOEL A. HIRSCH, DDS
Clinical Associate Professor, Advanced
Education Program in Prosthodontics,
Department of Prosthodontics, College of
Dentistry, New York University; Private
Practice, New York, New York

OLE T. JENSEN, DDS, MS
Adjunct Professor, School of Dentistry,
University of Utah, Salt Lake City, Utah

BACH LE, DDS, MD, FICD, FACD
Clinical Associate Professor, Department of
Oral and Maxillofacial Surgery, The Herman
Ostrow School of Dentistry of USC,
Los Angeles County/USC Medical Center,
Los Angeles, California

KATINA NGUYEN, DDS
Philip J. Boyne and Peter Geistlich Research
Fellow, Department of Oral and Maxillofacial
Surgery, Loma Linda University, Loma Linda,
California

BRADY NIELSEN, DDS
Chief Resident, Department of Oral and
Maxillofacial Surgery, The Herman Ostrow
School of Dentistry of USC, Los Angeles
County/USC Medical Center, Los Angeles,
California

RICARDO TRINDADE, DDS
PhD Student, Department of Prosthodontics,
Faculty of Odontology, Malmö University,
Malmö, Sweden

CHRISTOPHER T. VOGEL, DDS
Department of Oral and Maxillofacial Surgery,
University of Missouri-Kansas City, Kansas
City, Missouri

ANN WENNERBERG, DDS, PhD
Department of Prosthodontics, Faculty of
Odontology, Malmö University, Malmö,
Sweden

GEORGE SHELBY WHITE, DDS, FACP
Associate Clinical Professor, Director, Division
of Prosthodontics, Columbia University College
of Dental Medicine, New York, New York

Contents

will be needed. Many options for treatment of alveolar ridge defects are available, including varying surgical techniques as well as bone graft options.

Maxillary Sinus Bone Augmentation Techniques

245

Vincent Carrao and Isabelle DeMatteis

Maxillary sinus expansion and atrophy can be difficult to overcome for patients who require functional dental prostheses. One solution for this problem is sinus augmentation and implant placement. Patients are evaluated and diagnosis is ascertained, leading to development of a treatment plan and surgical strategy. The surgeon decides on a surgical technique and grafting material, based on ultimate success, stability, and function as they relate to the goals. Complications can occur during an operation or during the postoperative healing phase. Dealing with these complications can be challenging; however, solving these problems positively affects the overall outcome and success.

Prosthodontic Considerations in Post-cancer Reconstructions

255

Piriya Boonsiriphant, Joel A. Hirsch, Alex M. Greenberg, and Eric M. Genden

The restoration of function after oncologic surgery of the oral cavity constitutes one of the major challenges facing head and neck oncology. Within the general objective of securing esthetic as well as functional reconstructions, dental rehabilitation is crucial for achieving a good outcome. Adequate dental rehabilitation allows the patient to chew food and considerably improves speech and swallowing. These reconstructions will be driven biologically or prosthodontically following surgical design and outcome.

Treatment of the Edentulous Patient

265

George Shelby White

For decades, the edentulous population has been unrecognized in its need to be treated in an effective manner. The debilitating condition affects quality of life. Implants have provided a strategy for developing a standard of care. The McGill consensus statement provided evidence that 2 implants supporting a mandibular overdenture should be the first choice in the treatment of edentulism. Success in implementing this standard of care into an institution's curriculum depends on a close collaboration between the surgeon and the restoring dentist and an understanding of biomechanics and bone biology.

Dental Extraction, Immediate Placement of Dental Implants, and Immediate Function

273

Ole T. Jensen

Immediate function requires adequate implant stability and prosthetic stability, particularly when multiple implants are loaded. Factors to consider for immediate implants into extraction sites are thickness of socket walls, thickness of gingival drape, optimal position of the implant, and patient factors such as hygiene and smoking cessation.

Esthetic Implant Site Development

283

Bach Le and Brady Nielsen

Bony support is critical for creating and maintaining esthetic and natural-appearing peri-implant soft tissue profiles. A variety of techniques has been shown to be effective for augmenting bone and soft tissue. Ideal implant position and angulation is critical for a natural-appearing outcome. Achieving an ideal esthetic result in the compromised site is often elusive and in many cases, impossible. This article reviews techniques available for esthetic implant site development. A review of the recent literature discovers the most effective techniques for achieving esthetic results.

This article discusses surgical complications associated with the placement of dental implants, specifically focusing on how they occur (etiology), as well as their management and prevention. Dental implant surgical complications can be classified into those of hard and soft tissues. In general, complications can be avoided with thorough preoperative treatment planning and proper surgical technique.

Oral and maxillofacial surgeons now have extraordinary imaging, software planning, and guide fabrication technologies at their disposal to aid in their case selection, clinical decision making, and surgical procedures for dental implant placement. Cone beam CT has opened a new era of office-based diagnostic capability and responsibility. Improved clinical experiences and evidence-based superior outcomes can be provided with confidence to patients when CT-guided dental implant surgery is used.

ORAL AND MAXILLOFACIAL SURGERY CLINICS OF NORTH AMERICA

THE CLINICS ARE NOW AVAILABLE ONLINE!
Access your subscription at:
www.theclinics.com

Preface
Dental Implants and Evolving Discipline

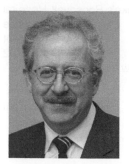

Alex M. Greenberg, DDS
Editor

Modern dental implantology begins with the work of Professor Per-Ingvar Brånemark (1929-2014) at the University of Gothenburg, Sweden, and Professor André Schroeder (1918-2004) at the University of Bern, Switzerland. Professor Brånemark was the first to observe that titanium had the unique property of developing a permanent attachment to bone, which he termed "osseointegration." From this observation, he then had the further understanding that titanium could be utilized as a material for permanent dental implants. At the Toronto Conference on Osseointegration in Clinical Dentistry in 1982, Professor Brånemark gave his landmark presentation that convinced dentists that a new era had dawned for dental implants, which became rapidly adopted as a new method of root form screws. Many other individuals contributed further to the development of modern dental implants, including Professor Andre Schroeder, who published in 1976 early histological evidence of dental implant osseointegration and collaborated with Dr Fritz Straumann of Waldenburg, Switzerland to develop improved dental implant designs. Continued scientific research into the basic science of bone biology, dental implant metal surfaces, and metallurgy has allowed new dental implant developments. Building on the refinements of dental implants themselves were new developments in bone augmentation through various biomaterials and surgical grafting techniques. Guided tissue regeneration, first reported by Professor Anthony Melcher in 1976, and was initially performed with nonresorbable, and then later with resorbable membranes, revolutionized the ability of practitioners to reconstruct the various bony defects that commonly presented in which implants could not be placed. The development of the indirect and direct sinus lift bone graft by Dr Oscar Hilt Tatum in 1974 opened further frontiers for those suffering from posterior maxillary edentulism. New biomaterials such as rhBMP-2 further improved the possibilities for complex bone graft augmentation of alveolar ridges and reducing the need for major bone grafting. The recent development of office-based cone beam CT imaging technologies and CT-guided surgery, new surgical and prosthetic biomaterials, improved dental implants, and other clinical innovations allow clinicians to further advance their ability to provide patients with partial and total edentulism with a greater variety of simple to complex advanced treatment options. As the field of dental implants has undergone these new developments, it is important for practitioners to have a better clinical and scientific understanding of complications and their management.

Oral Maxillofacial Surg Clin N Am 27 (2015) ix–x
http://dx.doi.org/10.1016/j.coms.2015.03.001
1042-3699/15/$ – see front matter © 2015 Published by Elsevier Inc.

We are fortunate that this issue of *Oral and Maxillofacial Surgery Clinics of North America* brings together so many outstanding articles in a cohesive presentation of the latest clinical and scientific understanding that we have of dental implants. I am deeply grateful to the many authors for their essential contributions and to the editorial staff at Elsevier for their support of this issue.

Dental implantology is truly "an evolving discipline," as seen by the remarkable advances since the early work of Professors Brånemark, Schroeder, and many others. This issue should be a valuable asset to Oral and Maxillofacial Surgeons in their clinical dental implant practice.

Alex M. Greenberg, DDS
Oral and Maxillofacial Surgery
Columbia University College of Dental Medicine
630 W 168th st, New York, NY 10032, USA

The New York Presbyterian Hospital
The Mount Sinai Hospital
The Mount Sinai Beth Israel Hospital
The Mount Sinai St. Luke's Roosevelt Hospital
Private Practice
18 East 48th Street
Suite 1702
New York, NY 10017, USA

E-mail address:
nycimplant@aol.com

Current Concepts for the Biological Basis of Dental Implants

Foreign Body Equilibrium and Osseointegration Dynamics

Ricardo Trindade, DDS[a], Tomas Albrektsson, MD, PhD, RCPSG[a,b], Ann Wennerberg, DDS, PhD[a,*]

KEYWORDS

- Implants • Osseointegration • Foreign body reaction

KEY POINTS

- Bone as a complex and multifunctional tissue is an important factor in osseointegration.
- Implant protein adsorption and the immune system are key determinants.
- Foreign body equilibriumis is same as a successful osseointegration
- Osseointegration is a dynamic process results from a complex set of reactions.
- Several host mechanisms and pathways interact to allow the integration of the implant in the host tissues, namely bone and oral mucosa.

INTRODUCTION

It has long been established that successful osseointegration, with direct bone apposition onto the surface of the implant,[1] is the 1 key event that allows millions of implants to successfully help in replacing inevitably lost teeth every year.

One must have an individualistic approach to patients in need of implants, if biology is to be considered; the genetic basis of individuals plays a more important role than might be perceived initially, which has been demonstrated by studies that link early periimplant marginal bone loss to certain genetic polymorphisms of cytokines such as interleukin (IL)-1β,[2,3] whereas habits such as smoking and alcohol consumption, or the intake of medicines for certain diseases, are thought to have an effect on the human body mechanisms that guide the dental implant–host relationship.

Upon insertion, implanted materials are coated rapidly with blood and interstitial fluids' proteins that get adsorbed onto the surface; 1 hypothesis is that it is to this adsorbed layer that cells primarily respond and not to the surface itself, although it is clear that such cell surface interaction is pivotal for cell survival, growth, and differentiation.[4]

Clearly, the importance of the pristine surface is substantial because one particular surface may produce a severely different effect on host proteins when compared with another surface, which may in turn result in a profound difference regarding the subsequent tissue formation around the implant.

The immune system, previously overlooked by many researchers, is believed to play a decisive role in the biological mechanisms that determine the fate of any implant placed within living tissues.[5,6] This means an important shift in paradigm is taking place, where biomaterials are perceived

[a] Department of Prosthodontics, Faculty of Odontology, Malmö University, Carl Gustavsväg 34, 214 21 Malmö, Sweden; [b] Department of Biomaterials, Sahlgrenska Academy, Gothenburg University, Arvid Wallgrens backe 20, 413 46 Gothenburg, Sweden
* Corresponding author.
E-mail address: ann.wennerberg@mah.se

Oral Maxillofacial Surg Clin N Am 27 (2015) 175–183
http://dx.doi.org/10.1016/j.coms.2015.01.004

as immunomodulatory rather than inert bodies, with huge consequences for implant dentistry and other biomedical applications.

The focus is currently changing regarding how host molecules and cells first interact through complex mechanisms when reacting to an invading foreign entity with particular chemistry, surface characteristics (that might have been manipulated or not in an attempt to achieve an improved outcome), and macroscopic design for favorable load distribution. All such factors play an essential role on the immediate and long-term success of osseointegration at the cellular level and is explored in this article.

TISSUE CHARACTERISTICS

To understand the biological basis of osseointegration, one has to understand the 2 main sides of the implant–host interaction: the tissue characteristics and the biomaterial characteristics. This article addresses the osseous tissue characteristics, as well as the potential role of soft tissues in dental implant's osseointegration.

Bone as an Immune and Endocrine Organ

The bone marrow is known to be a hematopoietic organ. Some authors also consider bone as an immunity regulatory organ, given the presence of dendritic cells (DCs), regulatory and conventional T cells, B cells, neutrophils, and mesenchymal stem cells, which elicit a role in regulating body wide immune reactions.[7]

Furthermore, besides being the target of hormones, bone also seems to function as an endocrine organ, as recent evidence suggests that 2 bone-derived factors can work as hormones:

a. Fibroblast growth factor 23 is produced by osteocytes in bone and inhibits hydroxylation of vitamin D and promotes phosphorous excretion in the kidney
b. Osteocalcin, a frequently assayed mediator in osseointegration studies, is also considered a hormone produced by bone osteoblasts acting distantly on pancreatic β cells to stimulate insulin production, on muscle cells inducing glucose uptake and on adipocytes to increase adiponectin production.[8]

Therefore, bone is a complex living tissue:

a. With its calcium homeostasis function
b. Functioning as an organ with the responsibility of producing hematopoietic cell lineages
c. Populated by immune cells that regulate inflammation and the immune system

d. Has an endocrine function through the production of mediators that work not only in a paracrine fashion, but that in reality are hormones that have an effect on distant organs and tissues.

Hence, bone-born implants are placed in a complex tissue (many functions of which were unknown until recently) that can be affected potentially by certain implant material characteristics. Osseointegration of implant devices may also be affected potentially by these cells and mediators that populate the osseous tissue.

Bone Cells

Bone remodeling results primarily from the coupled function of 2 of the bone cells, which are interdependent:

a. Osteoblasts (bone-forming cells)
b. Osteoclasts (bone-resorbing cells).

Another important notion is the organization of these cells in basic multicellular units (BMU), which perform the remodeling task.[9] The fine balance between bone formation and bone resorption is controlled by an intricate web of pathways that act on and from the BMU; depending on the stimuli, the result will be either bone growth or loss. Regulation of bone homeostasis and remodeling is known to also involve immune cells, such as B and T lymphocytes, whereas cells known as osteomacs (macrophages present in the bone in close connection with osteoblasts) have been demonstrated, in vitro and in vivo, to regulate the osteoblastic mineralization activity.[9] From an osseointegration point of view, the role of BMUs in a biomaterial context has not yet been entirely understood.

Further studies are also needed on how different stimuli, such as certain drugs, diseases, or local strains from an implant may affect the BMU, and how this may prevent the desired bone quantity and quality and thus hinder the successful clinical application of an implant.[10]

As for the remaining bone cell type, osteocytes, a recent publication has reported on the direct contact between these cells' dendrites and the implant surface, after an 8-week osseointegration period in an in vivo model. From this viewpoint, and considering that osteocytes are important cell homeostasis regulators and may act as mechanosensors, further studies are needed regarding the role of these cells in long term osseointegration maintenance.[11]

Cellular and Molecular Basis of Osseointegration

Osseointegration is a dynamic process that results from a complex set of reactions, where several host mechanisms and pathways interact to allow the integration of the implant in the host tissues, namely bone and oral mucosa. Once the implant material is perceived in the described biological context, it is easier to understand the reactions that potentially take place at the implant–tissue interface.

In implant dentistry, the literature has focused over the years on describing osseointegration from a purely wound healing point of view. Material science, nevertheless, has been describing the participation of the immune system in the relationship of biomaterials with host tissues for a few decades now. There is no doubt that the successful integration of implants, regardless of tissue type, is driven by inflammatory processes. In fact, without inflammation, integration in the tissues may not even take place. To correctly understand the osseointegration of dental implants, a deeply embedded concept must be challenged. In dental implant science, titanium and other materials being applied for the same purposes have so far been considered inert. However, some authors currently consider that implant materials, be those intraoral or extraoral implants, orthopedic implants or even bone substitutes, may instead be immunomodulatory.[12]

This change in concept raises 2 questions:

a. If a material is capable of modulating the immune system, what consequences may be expected?
b. In what manner is the immune system important to the bone and even the soft tissue response to dental implants?

First, biomaterials are unlikely to be inert when in contact with living tissues. This is because proteins are adsorbed instantly onto the surfaces of all foreign materials once these are implanted.[13] Protein adsorption is the first key for tissue integration with biomaterials, and this physicochemical property is set to influence the ensuing group of reactions, modulating the host response in its entirety. Protein adsorption consists, in general terms, of the unfolding of local host proteins when in contact with the biomaterial surface. This conformational change results in the exposure of potentially biologically active peptide units (epitopes) that can trigger a different set of host molecular and cellular responses, when compared with a situation where a biomaterial is absent.[14] Such resulting set of reactions may be beneficial or not to the patient.

Eaton and Tang and colleagues have worked on the relationship of protein adsorption with biomaterial integration and in 1 study found that

fibrinogen, a known important glucoprotein at surface interaction, behaves differently when adsorbed or denatured, when compared with the nonadsorbed, soluble form. Once adsorbed, fibrinogen exposes 2 previously hidden amino acid sequences P1 and P2, that function as epitopes and bind to phagocyte's integrin Mac-1 (CD11b/CD18) leading to a proinflammatory environment and modulating the host response to the biomaterial. Thrombin-mediated conversion of fibrinogen to fibrin also exposes the P1 and P2 epitopes, with similar consequences,[15] eliciting the participation of thrombotic events in the implant osseointegration events.

Protein adsorption is intimately related to the surface characteristics of the material, a feature that has been studied extensively. Surface topography, for instance, is known to be fundamental for improved osteoconduction of implant biomaterials,[16] playing a crucial role in the complex bone–implant interface reactions both at the microstructure and nanostructure levels.[17] Osseointegration of titanium implants depends on the cellular response to surface modifications and coatings,[18] which is intimately related with the protein adsorption pattern.[19]

Studies have focused mostly on the ability of the proteins adsorbed to promote the adhesion of osteoblasts,[20,21] and some authors have extended their interpretation to the benefit of avoiding the attachment of bacteria, in a so-called selective protein adsorption[22] through a process that avoids the adsorption of nonspecific proteins, affording a nonfouling surface to titanium, although it is not clear if such change of surface chemistry with peptides will negatively interfere with osseointegration.

Other studies have used implants coated with key proteins (eg, fibrinogen), assessing the biological response,[23,24] when compared with uncoated implants.

a. Fibrinogen seems to have a beneficial effect on tissue integration
b. Bougas and colleagues[25] have demonstrated in vitro that laminin induces a higher calcium-phosphate (CaP) deposition on the implant surfaces, even though the in vivo performance at the early osseointegration period was difficult to demonstrate at this initial stage of research.

Such mechanisms are yet to be understood and protein adsorption remains a controversial topic, especially when considering that it might be beneficial in some biomedical applications, whereas for others it could be detrimental (friend or foe?).

The doubts surrounding protein adsorption are:

a. Identifying the key proteins in the process
b. Whether some are unwanted
c. And especially to what extent should a protein unfold, because different degrees of linear conformation could possibly expose different peptide units, ending up in potentially different outcomes, some not necessarily beneficial for the implant integration with the tissues.

Evidently, more emphasis and importance is placed by the current text authors on the chemical and signaling ability of the protein adsorption phenomenon, although this cell adhesion facilitation is not discarded. In such a context, it is understood that the adsorption event is likely to influence the local immune response, by modulating the immune system components in reacting in a certain way. This process is what was referred to as immunomodulation.

IMMUNE SYSTEM AND TISSUE INTEGRATION

The immune system is thought to play a crucial role in biomaterial integration in host living tissues.
Several mechanisms are to be considered:

a. The normal healing mechanisms in response to the trauma caused by the surgical implant procedure that involve different cellular and molecular mechanisms, such as the coagulation system, the kinin system, platelets, fibroblasts, osteoblasts, and mesenchymal stem cells, among others[26]
b. An immune response that runs not only in parallel, but also interacting with the mechanisms in point (a), resulting in a complex network of reactions that dictate the long-term fate of the implant.[27]

It is believed that the host reaction to implants is regulated by innate immunity (the human body's nonspecific defense mechanisms, performed by the complement system, monocyte-macrophage cell lineages and B1-type lymphocytes),[6,28,29] although adaptive immunity (antigen-specific defense mechanisms, mediated by B or T lymphocytes) might also play a role in such a process.[30] After the protein adsorption phenomenon, the complement system is activated[5] and macrophages guide the inflammatory response to the biomaterial.[6]

Complement System

The complement system is part of the innate (nonspecific) immunity. It is composed by several plasma and cell membrane proteins that have the important task of distinguishing "self" from "nonself" entities, including foreign bodies,[31] participating in the direct or indirect (through activation of immune cells) elimination of threats to the human body.

Studies on biomaterials that are in direct contact with whole blood have reported on the role of the complement system, through its different known pathways, in guiding the host reaction to such biomedical applications.[31,32] Beside immune cells, like macrophages and lymphocytes, complement factors are also known to interact with osteoblasts under certain conditions, while also being able to induce osteoclastogenesis.[6] The complement system may, thus, have an important role in mediating implant–host interactions, such as the one leading to osseointegration.

Macrophages

Macrophages represent another important key in the osseointegration process. Macrophages are considered the sentry cells of the immune system; they work as a traffic roundabout where all immunologic and inflammatory reactions are controlled and guided.[29,30] This process is not understood entirely, but that is the center of attention for a considerable number of researchers integrating teams that focus on all aspects of health-related topics, including oncology, nutrition, atherosclerosis, and autoimmune diseases. They are also being studied and applied in cell therapy for the treatment of some diseases.[29]

Macrophages play an important role in the inflammatory balance, because they can assume rather different phenotypes that depend on local conditions:

a. M1 macrophages present the classical phagocytic and proinflammatory characteristics
b. M2 macrophages are involved in tissue repair and healing.[33]

Even more interesting is the versatility of macrophages, which adapt their phenotype to changes in the local environment.[6]

The role of macrophages in osseointegration is greater than previously expected. Basically, although neutrophils are recruited on the basis of a pure wound healing phenomena, macrophages are only recruited if a biomaterial is present[27]; when in the presence of foreign entities, macrophages further fuse into foreign body giant cells that are multinucleated giant cells formed to deal with larger targets.[34] These cells are found frequently on the surface of titanium oral implants[35] and justify the concept of osseointegration being a foreign body reaction,[5,6] because oral implants are in themselves foreign bodies. This concept was early realized by the German pathologist Karl Donath, who suggested such concept in a work published in 1992.[36]

Albrektsson and colleagues[5] introduced the concept of foreign body equilibrium:

a. Osseointegration is the result of a foreign body reaction that, with the right intensity in the inflammatory response, will balance itself out and allow for bone to grow on the implant surface
b. Similar to soft tissue implants, which end up encapsulated in poorly enervated and vascularized fibrous tissue, dental implants also become surrounded by condensed bone that is very poor in vascularization and enervation, the typical result of a foreign body reaction that has reached equilibrium[5]
c. The ongrown bone may be seen as a manner of shielding off the foreign entity from the tissues, that is, as a protective mechanism.

Lymphocytes

Lymphocytes interact with macrophages and also with bone cells, thus eliciting their participation in the osseointegration process.[12] The question is whether lymphocytes render an acquired immunity participation in the process or if it stays within the innate immunity boundaries. We also need to clarify whether these cells play a role in the buildup process that result in osseointegration or if only activated during the pathologic breakdown of osseointegration, leading to marginal bone loss.[6]

Marginal Bone Loss

In the same context, periimplant bone loss is the result of the immunologically led loss of the inflammatory balance. This concept is reinforced by the fact that osteoclasts, which are bone resorbing cells, can result from the fusion of macrophages[6,37]; however, some authors suggest that macrophages are themselves able to perform bone resorption.[38] It is not clear whether the bone loss seen and described as periimplantitis by Albrektsson and Isidor in 1994[39] is the result of bacterial colonization through the implant surrounding mucosa, despite this being the currently accepted theory in implant dentistry.

The mechanisms involved in such pathologic finding, for example, receptor activator nuclear factor-κB ligand (RANKL, which promotes macrophage fusion into foreign body giant cells and osteoclasts)[37] are also expressed in inflammatory pathologic conditions that do not result from infection, such as autoimmune diseases like rheumatoid arthritis[40] and in what is described in orthopedics as aseptic loosening,[41] where periimplant bone loss occurs in the absence of bacteria.

Marginal bone loss around oral implants is related to the implant type, clinical handling, and patient characteristics,[42] a trilogy that is difficult to couple to a disease such as periodontitis around teeth. The start of marginal bone loss around oral implants depends on disturbance of the foreign body equilibrium owing to the trilogy of factors and is characterized by recruitment of bone resorbing cells and gradual disappearance of bony support around implants. At this initial stage, a bacterial infection (the current definition of periimplantitis) is not likely, representing only a late complication of marginal bone resorption. In many cases, bone resorption may be active for years without developing periimplantitis, but with increasing time and loss of bony support, a secondary bacterial superinfection is gradually becoming a likely scenario; hence, periimplantitis may represent a complication to already ongoing bone resorption of an aseptic nature.

When bacterial colonization has finally set in, we may have a dual source of recruitment of bone resorbing cells, one of an aseptic and the other of a septic origin.[6,43,44] In other words, infection is not likely to be the initial trigger of bone resorption, but biomaterials may activate innate and/or adaptive immunity in a similar way to that of bacterial lipopolysaccharides. In fact, it has been suggested that the gradual development of periimplant bone loss may be based entirely on a foreign body reaction.[5,6]

Soft Tissues and Foreign Body Equilibrium

The soft tissue seal around dental implants is fundamental for the long-term success of osseointegrated dental implants. Mucosa, like skin, represents the first barrier and first line of defense against external aggressions against the human body. Langerhans cells are DCs that can be found in skin and mucosa (including the oral one)[45] and are known to represent the most peripheral outpost of the immune system.[46] Because these cells are antigen presenting and of mononuclear origin, like macrophages, a role in the foreign body reaction could be expected. Macrophages and their fusion into foreign body giant cells, as stated, are considered a hallmark of the foreign body reaction, although it is believed that a great part of the ensuing reactions to biomaterials are controlled by these cells[6] through inflammatory mediators and interactions with lymphocytes, fibroblasts (in soft tissues), and osteoblasts/osteoclasts (in hard tissues).

Myeloid DCs are equally considered important bridges between the innate and adaptive immune systems, playing a role in many inflammatory diseases through processes still not entirely understood,[47] eliciting a potential role for the foreign body reaction, a similar inflammatory process with immunologic characteristics. It has been suggested further that biomaterials are agonists for DCs maturation and influence the phenotype developed, with repercussions for the immune response guiding the foreign body reaction.[48]

An in vitro study has found that Langerhans cells in the oral mucosa are more effective in stimulating T cells than their skin counterparts.[49] In another in vitro study, the same authors concluded that this might be owing to a suppressive factor in the skin environment, although such a factor has not been identified.[50] Clarification is needed for such relationship between immune cells on the oral mucosa and biomaterials, and how this can affect the success of the treatment with implantable devices.

Psoriasis is an autoimmune disease and the differences in behavior of DCs in skin lesions of patients with such ailment have been addressed. It has been reported that there is an inflammatory dermal DC phenotype CD11c$^+$CD1c$^-$ in psoriatic skin lesion areas, when compared with a resident cutaneous DC phenotype is CD11c$^+$CD1$^+$; the inflammatory DCs express a higher amount of inflammatory mediators.[47]

It would be of interest to investigate whether different DC phenotypes exist in the soft tissue displaying periimplant disease in the oral mucosa and whether these patients have actually been diagnosed previously with any immunologic dyscrasia. Having said this, there is a lack of evidence that marginal bone resorption must be preceded by mucositis, as suggested by some clinical scientists.

Keratinocytes of the basal layer are responsible for the continued supply of differentiated cells for reepithelization.[51] It remains to be understood whether, after implant insertion of a transmucosal implant, the dynamic process of the soft tissue to reepithelize is maintained, or whether this ability is negatively affected under inflammatory conditions, such as those caused by the surgical procedure to place the implant or resulting from the mere long-term tissue contact with the biomaterial, representing an altered foreign body equilibrium.

Furthermore, inflammatory DC phenotypes produce inflammatory mediators, including tumor necrosis factor–related, apoptosis-inducing ligand, which could have a direct effect on keratinocytes and/or other skin cell types to promote disease pathogenesis.[47]

Another important aspect in the periimplant soft tissue equation is the basement membrane. In the skin, the basement membrane firmly attaches the epidermis to the dermis and in the mucosa it connects the epithelium to the underlying connective tissue. Problems at the basement membrane form the basis of pathologies like epidermolysis bullosa, which can affect individuals in a hereditary fashion, both at the mucosal and skin level, causing clinical fragility and blistering of these structures.[52] An in vitro study suggests that production of the protein components (different kinds of collagen, integrins, laminin, etc) depends on keratinocytes and fibroblasts.[52]

When considering implant biomaterials, periimplant soft tissue loss or unfavorable transformation could be related hypothetically to changes at the basement membrane that can result from alterations in fibroblasts, keratinocytes, collagen, laminin, integrin, and other relevant factors, especially those with inflammatory and/or immunologic roles, that could ultimately influence the foreign body reaction process guiding the implant–tissue integration. Hence, the soft tissue integration is also likely to depend on a foreign body type of reaction and is intimately related to the material surface characteristics and composition. Integrity can be threatened equally by potentially pathologic conditions independent of bacterial colonization.

OSSEOINTEGRATION DYNAMICS

Following this explanation, osseointegration seems to depend not on a single pathway, but on a build-up system, whereas marginal bone loss depends on a breakdown system of reactions.[6] These systems characterize the dynamic nature of osseointegration; we now term these systems of reactions osseointegration dynamics (**Fig. 1**), which ensures that all parts considered are valued and taken into account. Osseointegration dynamics brings other challenges. It emphasizes the nonperennial nature of oral implants osseointegration, meaning that implants have to be followed, with clinicians paying special attention to overload situations or initial inflammatory conditions that need prompt intervention, because these tend to be asymptomatic, if displaying initial bone resorption.

Osseointegration dynamics relates to the in vivo lifetime of the implant and is intimately related to long-term clinical success. It also leaves open doors to the development of different strategies to deal with periimplant pathology, and it motivates the development of better, more predictable, faster healing dental implants, which can only be achieved with a thorough understanding of osseointegration biology.

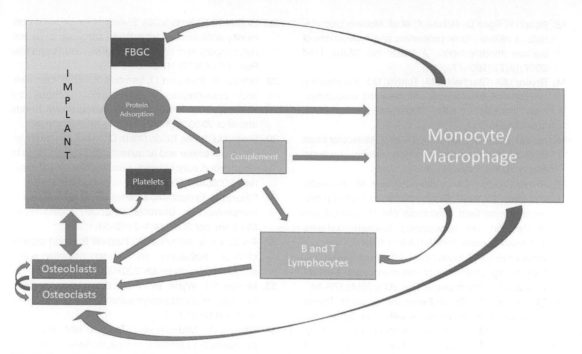

Fig. 1. Hypothetical model for osseointegration dynamics. FBGC, foreign body giant cells.

SUMMARY

Understanding the biology behind implant dentistry is of tremendous importance, because it opens the door to what should guide the development of solutions in the field: putting aside heuristic methods and replace them by methods that produce solutions to achieve a specific biological goal. It is obvious that trial and error will always be a part of science, as it, in its very essence, proposes to explore the unknown. But understanding biology is as important for scientists aiming at developing ever more predictable dental implant solutions as it is for clinicians upon deciding what is best for their patients, whether regarding a technique, a material or a whole treatment protocol.

REFERENCES

1. Albrektsson T, Branemark PI, Hansson HA, et al. Osseointegrated titanium implants. Requirements for ensuring a long-lasting, direct bone-to-implant anchorage in man. Acta Orthop Scand 1981;52(2): 155–70.

2. Lin Y, Huang P, Lu X, et al. The relationship between IL-1 gene polymorphism and marginal bone boss around dental implants. J Oral Maxillofac Surg 2007;65(11):2340–4.

3. Shimpuku H, Nosaka Y, Kawamura T, et al. Genetic polymorphisms of the interleukin-1 gene and early marginal bone loss around endosseous dental implants. Clin Oral Implants Res 2003;14(4):423–9.

4. Tang L, Hu W. Molecular determinants of biocompatibility. Expert Rev Med Devices 2005;2(4):493–500.

5. Albrektsson T, Dahlin C, Jemt T, et al. Is marginal bone loss around oral implants the result of a provoked foreign body reaction? Clin Implant Dent Relat Res 2014;16(2):155–65.

6. Trindade R, Albrektsson T, Tengvall P, et al. Foreign body reaction to biomaterials: on mechanisms for build-up and breakdown of osseointegration. Clin Implant Dent Relat Res 2014. [Epub ahead of print].

7. Zhao E, Xu H, Wang L, et al. Bone marrow and the control of immunity. Cell Mol Immunol 2012;9:11–9.

8. Fukumoto S, Martin TJ. Bone as an endocrine organ. Trends Endocrinol Metab 2009;20(5):230–6.

9. Kular J, Tickner J, Chim SM, et al. An overview of the regulation of bone remodelling at the cellular level. Clin Biochem 2012;45(12):863–73.

10. Frost HM. A brief review for orthopedic surgeons: fatigue damage (microdamage) in bone (its determinants and clinical implications). J Orthop Sci 1998; 3(5):272–81.

11. Du Z, Ivanovski S, Hamlet SM, et al. The ultrastructural relationship between osteocytes and dental implants following osseointegration. Clin Implant Dent Relat Res 2014. http://dx.doi.org/10.1111/cid.12257.

12. Chen Z, Wu C, Gu W, et al. Osteogenic differentiation of bone marrow MSCs by β-tricalcium phosphate stimulating macrophages via BMP2 signalling pathway. Biomaterials 2014;35(5):1507–18.

13. Roach P, Eglin D, Rohde K, et al. Modern biomaterials: a review - bulk properties and implications of surface modifications. J Mater Sci Mater Med 2007;18(7):1263–77.

14. Bryers JD, Giachelli CM, Ratner BD. Engineering biomaterials to integrate and heal: the biocompatibility paradigm shifts. Biotechnol Bioeng 2012; 109(8):1898–911.

15. Hu WJ, Eaton JW, Ugarova TP, et al. Molecular basis of biomaterial-mediated foreign body reactions. Blood 2001;98(4):1231–8.

16. Rivera-Chacon DM, Alvarado-Velez M, Acevedo-Morantes CY, et al. Fibronectin and vitronectin promote human fetal osteoblast cell attachment and proliferation on nanoporous titanium surfaces. J Biomed Nanotechnol 2013;9(6):1092–7.

17. Wennerberg A, Albrektsson T. Effects of titanium surface topography on bone integration: a systematic review. Clin Oral Implants Res 2009;20(4):172–84.

18. Mozumder MS, Zhu J, Perinpanayagam H. Titania-polymeric powder coatings with nano-topography support enhanced human mesenchymal cell responses. J Biomed Mater Res A 2012;100(10): 2695–709.

19. Boyd AR, Burke GA, Duffy H, et al. Sputter deposited bioceramic coatings: surface characterisation and initial protein adsorption studies using surface-MALDI-MS. J Mater Sci Mater Med 2011;22(1):71–84.

20. Buchanan LA, El-Ghannam A. Effect of bioactive glass crystallization on the conformation and bioactivity of adsorbed proteins. J Biomed Mater Res A 2010;93(2):537–46.

21. Divya Rani VV, Manzoor K, Menon D, et al. The design of novel nanostructures on titanium by solution chemistry for an improved osteoblast response. Nanotechnology 2009;20(19):195101.

22. Khoo X, Hamilton P, O'Toole GA, et al. Directed assembly of PEGylated-peptide coatings for infection-resistant titanium metal. J Am Chem Soc 2009; 131(31):10992–7.

23. Jimbo R, Sawase T, Shibata Y, et al. Enhanced osseointegration by the chemotactic activity of plasma fibronectin for cellular fibronectin positive cells. Biomaterials 2007;28(24):3469–77.

24. Tang L, Eaton JW. Fibrin(ogen) mediates acute inflammatory responses to biomaterials. J Exp Med 1993;178(6):2147–56.

25. Bougas K. On the influence of biochemical coating on implant bone incorporation [PhD Thesis]. Sweden: Department of Prosthodontics, Faculty of Odontology, Malmö University; 2012.

26. Anderson JM, Rodriguez A, Chang DT. Foreign body reaction to biomaterials. Semin Immunol 2008;20(2):86–100.

27. Jones KS. Effects of biomaterial-induced inflammation on fibrosis and rejection. Semin Immunol 2008; 20(2):130–6.

28. Ekdahl KN, Lambris JD, Elwing H, et al. Innate immunity activation on biomaterial surfaces: a mechanistic model and coping strategies. Adv Drug Deliv Rev 2011;63(12):1042–50.

29. Nilsson B, Korsgren O, Lambris JD, et al. Can cells and biomaterials in therapeutic medicine be shielded from innate immune recognition? Trends Immunol 2010;31(1):32–8.

30. Smith MJ, White KL Jr, Smith DC, et al. In vitro evaluations of innate and acquired immune responses to electrospun polydioxanone-elastin blends. Biomaterials 2009;30(2):149–59.

31. Nilsson B, Ekdahl KN, Mollnes TE, et al. The role of complement in biomaterial-induced inflammation. Mol Immunol 2007;44(1–3):82–94.

32. Arvidsson S, Askendal A, Tengvall P. Blood plasma contact activation on silicon, titanium and aluminium. Biomaterials 2007;28(7):1346–54.

33. Murray PJ, Wynn TA. Protective and pathogenic functions of macrophage subsets. Nat Rev Immunol 2011;11(11):723–37.

34. Moreno JL, Mikhailenko I, Tondravi MM, et al. IL-4 promotes the formation of multinucleated giant cells from macrophage precursors by a STAT6-dependent, homotypic mechanism: contribution of E-cadherin. J Leukoc Biol 2007;82(6):1542–53.

35. Khan UA, Hashimi SM, Khan S, et al. Differential expression of chemokines, chemokine receptors and proteinases by foreign body giant cells (FBGCs) and osteoclasts. J Cell Biochem 2014; 115:1290–8.

36. Donath K, Donath K, Laass M, et al. The histopathology of different foreign-body reactions in oral soft tissue and bone tissue. Virchows Arch A Pathol Anat Histopathol 1992;420(2):131–7.

37. Yagi M, Miyamoto T, Sawatani Y, et al. DC-STAMP is essential for cell-cell fusion in osteoclasts and foreign body giant cells. J Exp Med 2005;202(3): 345–51.

38. Tamaki Y, Sasaki K, Sasaki A, et al. Enhanced osteolytic potential of monocytes/macrophages derived from bone marrow after particle stimulation. J Biomed Mater Res B Appl Biomater 2008;84(1):191–204.

39. Albrektsson T, Isidor F. Consensus report of session IV. In: Lang NP, Karring T, editors. Proceedings of the First European Workshop on Periodontology. London: Quintessence; 1994. p. 365–9.

40. Haynes DR, Crotti TN, Loric M, et al. Osteoprotegerin and receptor activator of nuclear factor kappaB ligand (RANKL) regulate osteoclast formation by cells in the human rheumatoid arthritis joint. Rheumatology 2001;40(6):623–30.

41. Crotti TN, Smith MD, Findlay DM, et al. Factors regulating osteoclast formation in human tissues adjacent to peri-implant bone loss: expression of receptor activator NFκB, RANK ligand and osteoprotegerin. Biomaterials 2004;25(4):565–73.

42. Chrcanovic BR, Albrektsson T, Wennerberg A. Reasons for failures of oral implants. J Oral Rehabil 2014;41(6):443–76.

43. Ujiie Y, Todescan R, Davies JE. Peri-implant crestal bone loss: a putative mechanism. Int J Dent 2012; 2012:742439.

44. Higgins DM, Basaraba RJ, Hohnbaum AC, et al. Localized immunosuppressive environment in the foreign body response to implanted biomaterials. Am J Pathol 2009;175(1):161–70.

45. Barrett AW, Cruchley AT, Williams DM. Oral mucosal Langerhans' cells. Crit Rev Oral Biol Med 1996;7(1): 36–58.

46. Cutler CW, Jotwani R. Dendritic cells at the oral mucosal interface. J Dent Res 2006;85(8):678–89.

47. Zaba LC, Fuentes-Duculan J, Eungdamrong NJ, et al. Identification of TNF-related apoptosis-inducing ligand and other molecules that distinguish inflammatory from resident dendritic cells in patients with psoriasis. J Allergy Clin Immunol 2010;125(6): 1261–8.

48. Babensee JE. Interaction of dendritic cells with biomaterials. Semin Immunol 2008;20(2):101–8.

49. Hasséus B, Jontell M, Bergenholtz G, et al. Langerhans cells from human oral epithelium are more effective at stimulating allogeneic T cells in vitro than Langerhans cells from skin. Clin Exp Immunol 2004;136(3):483–9.

50. Hasséus B, Jontell M, Bergenholtz G, et al. T-cell costimulatory capacity of oral and skin epithelial cells in vitro: presence of suppressive activity in supernatants from skin epithelial cell cultures. Eur J Oral Sci 2004;112(1):48–54.

51. Mazlyzam AL, Aminuddin BS, Fuzina NH, et al. Mazlyzam reconstruction of living bilayer human skin equivalent utilizing human fibrin as a scaffold. Burns 2007;33(3):355–63.

52. Wang TW, Sun JS, Huang YC, et al. Skin basement membrane and extracellular matrix proteins characterization and quantification by real time RT-PCR. Biomaterials 2006;27(29):5059–68.

Cone Beam Computed Tomography Scanning and Diagnosis for Dental Implants

Alex M. Greenberg, DDS[a,b,]*

KEYWORDS

- CBCT • Oral and maxillofacial surgery • Dental implants

KEY POINTS

- CBCT has become an important new technology for oral and maxillofacial surgery practitioners.
- CBCT provides improved office-based diagnostic capability and applications for surgical procedures, such as CT guidance through the use of computer-generated drill guides.
- A thorough knowledge of the basic science of CBCT as well as the ability to interpret the images correctly and thoroughly is essential to current practice.

Recent advances in cone beam computed tomography (CBCT) have made office-based CBCT scanners affordable for oral and maxillofacial surgeons who now use this cross-sectional imaging technology on a daily basis for a wide variety of clinical problems.[1–4] CBCT is a form of helical CT scanning that has the advantage of providing higher-level bone imaging in a dental setting at a significantly lowered dosage of radiation.[5] Radiation dosage in dental offices has been a topic of recent controversy in the public media, and indications for CBCT use should follow the as low as reasonably achievable (ALARA) principle.[6] This is especially important with regard to use in children.[7] Aside from the use of CBCT for the examination of impacted teeth,[8,9] supernumerary teeth,[10] detection of dental fractures,[11] maxillary sinus anatomy,[12] mandibular canals,[13] endodontic lesions, extra root canals, caries and periodontal lesions,[14] temporomandibular joint (TMJ),[15,16] skeletal jaw deformities,[17] orthodontics,[18,19]

acquired deformities and reconstruction,[20] oral and maxillofacial trauma,[21] pathology,[22,23] and airway,[24] it is also used for dental implants.[4,25–29] Office-based CBCT has the further advantage of being used for dental implant treatment planning and CT-guided dental implant placement. CT-guided dental implant surgery through the use of surgical drill guides[30–36] allows precise dental implant placement trajectories, depth control, minimally invasive flapless procedures, and immediate temporary prosthesis placement.[30–36] Tomography is imaging by sections and is performed by the rotation of an x-ray source around the single axis of an anatomic structure. A sensor absorbs the x-ray opposite to the source during the movement of the device.[37] Developed in the 1930s by Alessandro Vallebona,[38] plain tomography was an improvement over plain radiography. Plain tomography allowed the removal of superimposed structures to be viewed as a 2-D slice. In dentistry, a form of conventional plain tomography

a Oral and Maxillofacial Surgery, Columbia University College of Dental Medicine, 630 W. 168th Street, New York, NY 10032, USA; b Private Practice Limited to Oral and Maxillofacial Surgery, 18 East 48th Street Suite 1702, New York, NY 10017, USA
* Corresponding author. Private Practice Limited to Oral and Maxillofacial Surgery, 18 East 48th Street Suite 1702, New York, NY 10017.
E-mail address: nycimplant@aol.com

Oral Maxillofacial Surg Clin N Am 27 (2015) 185–202
http://dx.doi.org/10.1016/j.coms.2015.01.002

that continues to be widely used is the orthopanto-gram or panoramic radiograph.[39] Panoramic radi-ography uses a variable depth of field or focal trough,[40] allowing anatomy at the target level to remain sharp while other structures are blurred in the background. The term, orthopantomogram, is used to describe the panoramic radiograph, because the teeth are displayed in the orthogonal plane. Modern tomography involves the taking of multiple projections of an anatomic region and feeding the data into a specialized reconstruction software algorithm for computer processing.[41,42]

CT scanning was first discovered by Godfrey Hounsfield in England in the early 1970s,[43–45] for which he and Allan MacLeod Cormack received a Nobel prize in 1979.[46,47] With the ability to use powerful computer algorithms that process data from a large number of sectional images, or slices, a 3-D image can be reconstructed. The CT scan became an improvement over the 2-D sectional imaging of plain tomography.[48] CT is based on projective geometry analysis of the slice data generated by rotation around a patient as a result of the synchronous movement of the x-ray source and the sensor.[49] The earliest cesium iodide scin-tillator sensors were positioned opposite to the x-ray source.

It was in the late 1960s that Hounsfield first conceptualized that it was possible to determine the inside contents of a box by taking radiographs from multiple angles around an object. Based on the basic principles of projective geometry, the first CT scanner was built with a moveable x-ray tube and sensor connected by a rod with the pivot point as the focus. The image created by the beam in the focal plane appeared sharper, with the images of the superimposed structures becoming background noise. Hounsfield designed a com-puter that could accept the 2-D x-ray data from different angles to create a series of images of the object formatted as slices. In 1971, the first commercial CT scanner was developed for scan-ning the brain, which was later followed by the full-body scanner. Hounsfield, in the process of creating the first CT scanner, was unaware at the time that Cormack had developed similar mathematical theorems. Robert Ledley, at Geor-getown University, later developed an improved full-body CT scanner that did not require a water tank.[50] Developed by Hounsfield at a research branch of EMI, a company best known for its music and recording business, CT was originally known as the EMI scan or the Beatles scan.[51–53] CAT, originally termed computed axial tomogra-phy, was shortened to CT scan. The CT sensors originally were made from cesium iodide and later replaced with ion chambers containing xenon gas

under high pressure. CT scanners create images as slices of patients in different planes through the use of tomographic reconstruction fast Fourier mathematical calculation algorithms based on a matrix memory whereby points of data are pro-cessed.[54] The algorithm of these calculations is based on the Radon transformation, named after Johann Radon's work in 1917.[55,56] The Radon transformation is the integral of a function over straight lines, and it represents the scattering of data obtained as the output of a cross-sectional tomographic scan (**Fig. 1**). The use of the inverse of the Radon transformation allows the recon-struction of the scattering data and is the mathe-matical foundation for CT.[57,58] This process is known as the back projection[59–62] and reverses the acquisition geometry, storing the results in another memory array. The Radon transformation is also known as a sinogram, which resembles the images of CT scans.[63] The Radon transform of a direct delta function is a distribution supported within the graph of a sine wave. Consequently, the Radon transform of numerous small objects can be seen graphically as blurred sine waves with different amplitudes and phases. The inverse of the Radon transform is thus used to reconstruct the original density from the scattering data (**Fig. 2**) and thereby forms the mathematical basis for CT reconstruction.[64]

The analysis of CT data can be performed by using 2 types of algorithm method: filtered back projection (FBP)[65] and iterative reconstruction (IR),[66] which both gives inexact results and repre-sents a compromise between computation time and accuracy. FBP requires less computation time compared with IR, but IR has decreased artifacts.[67]

In digital imaging, a single point in a raster image is known as a pixel (*pix* [pictures] and *el* [element]). The pixel is the smallest 2-D addressable element of a picture on a screen that can be controlled. Raster images are the basic images that appear on a computer monitor and, depending on the software, can be in high or low definition. A volu-metric pixel in 3-D space is known as a voxel (*vox* [volume] and *el* [element]), and when aggre-gated forms a 3-D volume-rendered image.

$$Rf(L) = \int_L f(x)\,|dx|.$$

Fig. 1. Radon's transform formula.

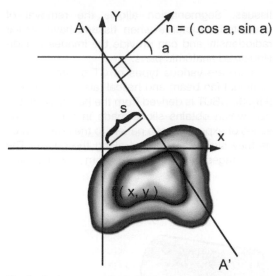

Fig. 2. Radon's transform back projection geometry.

Computer processing of CT scan data through the use of specialized algorithms allows a series of multiplanar reformatted voxel-based images to create a 3-D image of an anatomic structure.

Bone density is defined in CT scan images as Hounsfield units[68] (named after Hounsfield). Hounsfield units are a measurement of the difference between tissues from air to bone, in which disparities as little as 1% can be calculated (**Box 1**). Hounsfield units can be used to define bone mass but not quality.[69] It may be possible, however, to convert Hounsfield units into a useful classification of hard, normal, and soft, based on histomorphometric micro-CT.[70]

Turkyilmaz and colleagues[71] demonstrated measurements of Hounsfield units for each region of the jaw: posterior maxilla, 927; anterior maxilla, 721; anterior mandible, 708; and posterior mandible, 505.

Digital Imaging and Communications in Medicine (DICOM) is the format used for data created by CT and CBCT scanners.[71] The DICOM (National Electrical Manufacturers Association [NEMA] standard PS3 and International Organization for Standardization [ISO] standard 12052) format ensures that standard requirements for the format of an x-ray image file that in all instances must contain a patient identification. DICOM as a standard format enables the integration of servers, scanners, printers, workstations, and network hardware from different manufacturers into a picture archiving and communications system.[72,73]

Through a process called windowing, CT produces a volume of data that can be manipulated to demonstrate various bodily structures based on their radiodensity. Images generated are in the axial or transverse plane, orthogonal to the

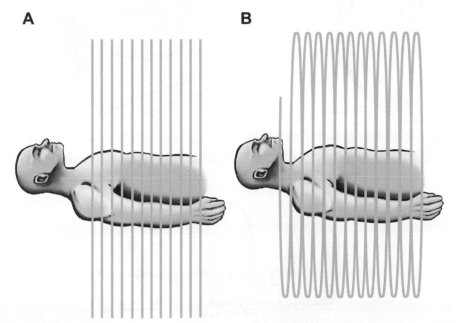

Fig. 3. (A) Fan beam CT and (B) helical (spiral) CT.

long axis of the body (ie, bone window or soft tissue window). CT scanners allow this volume of data to be reformatted in various planes or even as volumetric 3-D representations of hard or soft tissue highlighted structures. There are various 3-D volume rendering methods: shaded surface display, maximum intensity projection, and direct volume rendering.[74] Threshold density levels (ie, bone) can be formatted through surface rendering to create a 3-D image displayed on the monitor screen with different colors representing specific

tissues. Segmentation allows the removal of unwanted structures when tissues have similar radiodensity and can provide the images of individualized anatomic parts.

There are various types of CT scanners: conventional fan beam and helical (also called spiral) (**Fig. 3**). CBCT is derived from the helical CT scanner, which obtains slices made in a continuous series of exposures of a patient to the x-ray source as they slowly are moved along the gantry. The 3-D images are calculated from sophisticated

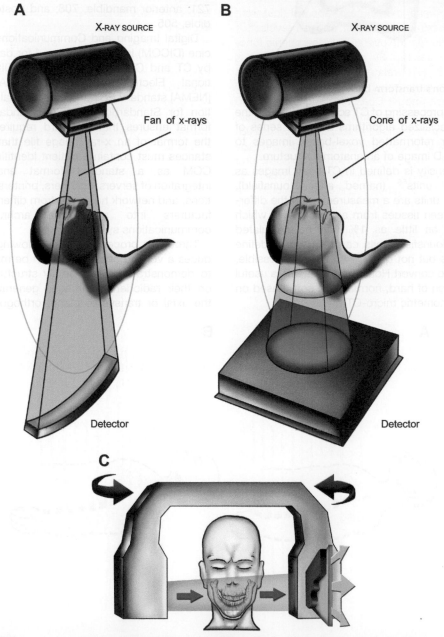

Fig. 4. (*A*) Fan beam CT scanner and (*B*) CBCT scanner. (*C*) FP CBCT scanner for sit-down or stand-up unit.

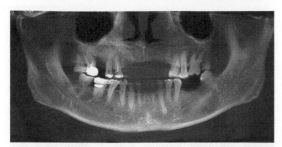

Fig. 5. Panoramic view.

algorithms of the scanner computer system that processes the series of individual slices. Currently, helical CT scanners obtain 64 or more slices per study. When a CBCT is performed, the x-ray beam is transmitted as a cone of x-rays that is detected as a volume of the patient registered on an area sensor instead of the multidirector array of helical CT scanners. Willi Kalendar developed the CBCT scanner[75–77] in the 1980s, which has become an affordable device for oral and maxillo-facial surgery practices. CBCT has dramatically reduced the radiation dosage for the scanning of patients in a dental setting compared with sending patients for medical helical CT scans (**Fig. 4**A and B). The CBCT uses newly developed less expensive x-ray tubes, improved area sensors, and the power of personal computer workstations to create smaller units for dental office settings (see **Fig. 4**C). There are 2 types of CBCT scanners: charge-coupled device (interline transfer [IT]-CCD), which uses a cesium gas–containing x-ray tube, and flat panel (FP), which contains an area sensor detector. The FP CBCT is similar to the conventional helical multidetector CT scanner except that the row of detectors has been replaced by cesium iodide scintillator crystals contained within the area sensor detector that converts the

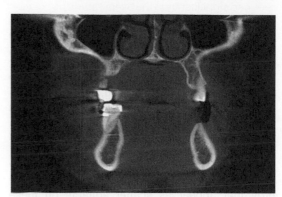

Fig. 7. Coronal view.

projection x-ray energy into light. The light is then converted into electrical signals by photodiodes for digital processing.[78] The FP units provide higher-resolution images at higher radiation doses, whereas the IT-CCD offers lower-dose radiation with less robust images.[79] The FP CBCT with its robust imaging capability can perform a dual scan that can acquire adequate data for manufacturing surgical guides from CT data alone. Some IT-CCD units are less capable of such features because of the lower radiation delivered. There are various types of units: sit-down, stand-up, prone, and mobile. Partial view units have also become increasingly popular because they provide sectional CT, which is at a further reduction of these already lowered radiation doses to patients.

The data from a single CBCT imaging procedure consist of multiple contiguous slices from 1 to 5 mm in thickness depending on the scanner, which contains approximately 300 individual images from a full field of view (FOV). The basic dental views are panoramic (**Fig. 5**), axial plane (**Fig. 6**), coronal plane (**Fig. 7**), sagittal plane (**Fig. 8**), lateral cephalometric (**Fig. 9**), TMJ

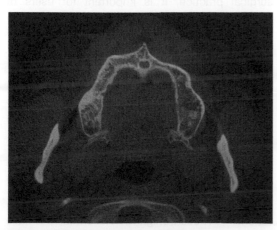

Fig. 6. Axial view.

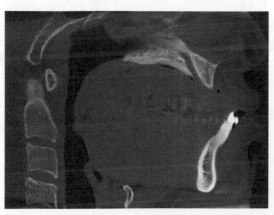

Fig. 8. Sagittal view.

(Fig. 10), and reformatted oblique sagittal (Fig. 11). CBCT volume rendering allows the reconstruction of 3-D images from multiplanar views (Fig. 12). Other benefits of CBCT from scanners with robust data are the ability to manufacture 3-D models by stereolithography, rapid printing, and rapid prototyping (Fig. 13). These models are built from data formatted as standard template library files (STL). CT scans of the jaws contain artifacts as a result of the presence of metallic dental restorations. The radiation that interacts with the high-density dental metallic restorations causes bursts of energy that appear as scatter artifacts on these different views (Fig. 14). Artifacts occur because the data values of these areas are higher than what the computer can process and appear as distortions.[80]

CBCT basic image acquisition is the lateral cephalometric image, also referred to as projection data. From the projection data, by using sophisticated computerized mathematical algorithms, a 3-D volumetric data set is generated. From the 3-D volumetric data set, primary reconstruction images are created in 3 orthogonal planes: axial, sagittal, and coronal.

There has been increased concern regarding the exposure of populations to CT scan radiation in the developed countries where large numbers of these studies have been performed. There is a direct correlation between the large increase in the number of available medical CT scanners and the high utilization of this imaging method. CT contributes to overall rise in radiation exposure to patients.[81] In 2007, there were 72 million studies in the United States.[82] There have been numerous reports regarding concern about CT imaging radiation causing increased cancer rates.[56–58] As a result of this widespread use, it is estimated[82–86] that as a result of the high utilization of CT scanners that there are negligible increases in cancer compared with those that result from background environmental radiation exposure. As a result of the radiation exposure from the approximately 600,000 abdominal and head CT examinations performed each year in children under 15 years of age in the United States, it is estimated that 500 of these individuals will die from cancer.[87]

Radiation dosages from plain dental radiography are well known, with Ludlow and colleagues[88] stating effective doses as full mouth exposures, 34.9 to 170.7 µSv; bitewing exposures, 5 µSv; and panoramic exposures, 14.2 to 24.3 µSv, which can be compared with background radiation dose from the environment of 3100 µSv.[89] CBCT radiation dosage has been studied by Roberts and colleagues[90] and found as full FOV, 206.2 µSv; 13-cm FOV, 133.9 µSv; 6-cm FOV high-resolution maxilla, 93.3 µSv; 5-cm FOV high-resolution mandible, 188.5 µSv; 6-cm standard mandible, 96.2 µSv; and 6-cm standard maxilla, 58.9 µSv. The FOV radiation has been noted to vary in different CBCT machines, from 51.7 to 193.4 µSv.[91] There has been concern regarding the lack of uniformity and evidence-based understanding of the actual radiation doses from various CBCT scanners.[91] Compared with CBCT, the radiation dose is substantially higher from a medical helical CT scan of the head (2000 µSv).[92] CBCT averages 5% to 10% of the radiation dose of a head medical helical CT scan. Depending on the CBCT scanner, the radiation dosage equivalent to a multiple of panoramic radiographs ranges, for a 12-inch FOV scan, from 15 to 78 µSv and, for a 9-inch FOV scan, from 5 to 33 µSv. The increased risk of cancer of radiation exposure from a full-body scan has been compared with the rate in atomic bomb survivors.[93]

In the routine course of oral and maxillofacial surgical practice, it is important for users of CBCT scanners to be completely familiar with all the different types of benign and malignant lesions that may be seen in these images. Benign dental pathology is seen as radiolucent, radiopaque, and mixed radiolucent and radiopaque lesions. Examples of radiolucent lesions are paradontal and dentigerous cysts[94–96] (Fig. 15), radicular cysts,[97] giant cell lesions,[98,99] traumatic[100] and aneurysmal bone cysts,[101] and vascular lesions. A majority of benign radiolucent lesions are unilocular with hyperostotic borders. Less frequent are the ameloblastomas (Fig. 16),[102,103] myxomas (Fig. 17),[104] odontogenic keratocyst or keratocystic odonogenic tumors (Fig. 18),[105] and giant cell lesions.[106] These benign radiolucent lesions have unilocular, multilocular, scalloped, honeycomb,

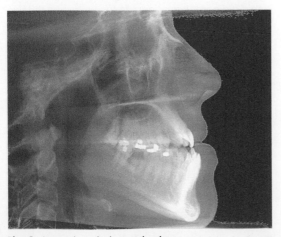
Fig. 9. Lateral cephalometric view.

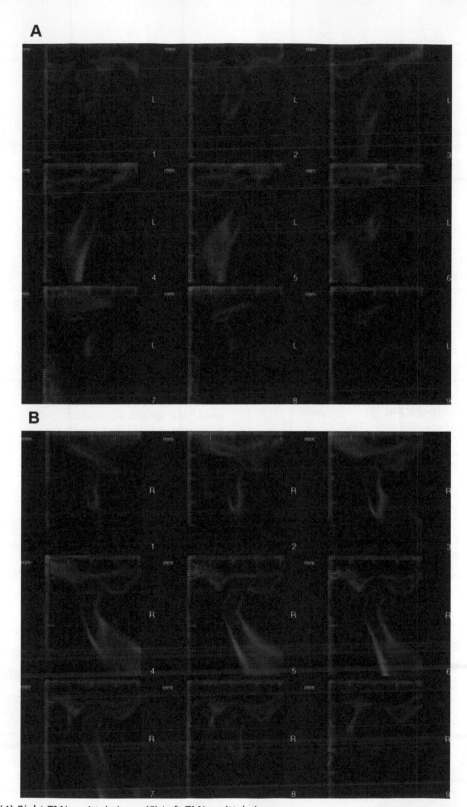

Fig. 10. (*A*) Right TMJ sagittal views. (*B*) Left TMJ sagittal views.

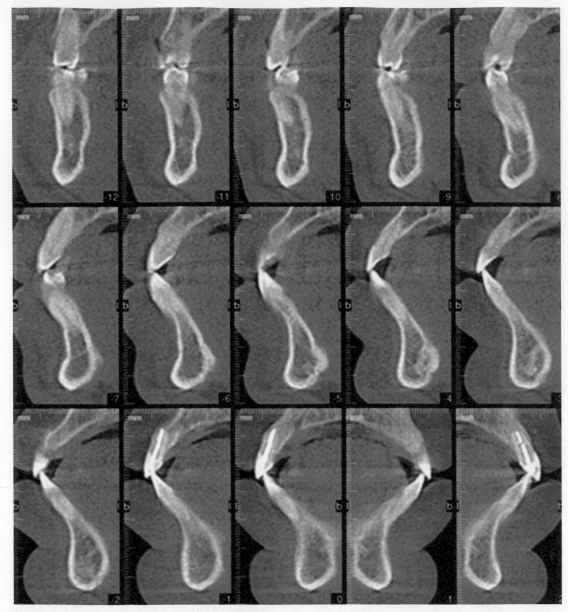

Fig. 11. Reformatted sagittal views of the mandible.

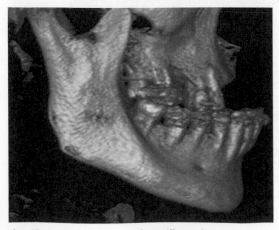

Fig. 12. 3-D lateral view of maxilla and mandible.

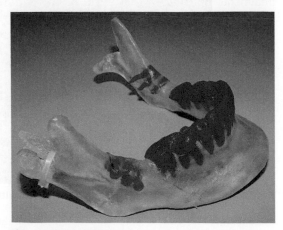

Fig. 13. Stereolithographic model of a mandible.

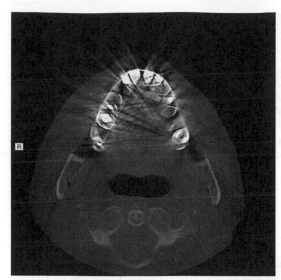

Fig. 14. Prominent artifacts secondary to maxillary fixed bridge metallic restorations.

more irregular, and destructive appearances. Decreased bone density, known as rarefaction, is seen usually as a precursor to periapical and periodontal pathology, which can be diffuse, for example, as in the early stage of an infection with loss of lamina dura prior to cyst formation. Radiopaque lesions may include pure osteomas,[107] exostoses (**Fig. 19**), cementomas or cemental dysplasia,[108,109] condensing osteitis,[110] odontomas, and supernumary teeth. Benign mixed radiopaque and radiolucent lesions include fibro-osseous[111] cement-ossifying lesions, such as cementossifying fibroma,[112] ossifying fibroma[113,114] adenomatoid odontogenic tumor (**Fig. 20**),[115] and Pindborg tumor.[116] Osteomyelitis is a mixed radiopaque and radiolucent lesion that is destructive in nature as a result of an infectious

process and can be similar to the appearance of malignancies (**Fig. 21**). Periosteal reaction[117] and finding of bone sclerosis[118] can be useful in differentiating osteomyelitis from malignancies, in addition to clinical and histopathological examination.

Malignant radiolucent lesions have irregular borders that are often diffuse in appearance, with destruction of the cortical bone borders, resorption of roots, tooth extrusion, tooth displacement, and, on serial studies, more rapid changes.[119] Examples are the purely radiolucent lesions, such as metastatic cancer, squamous cell carcinoma (**Fig. 22**), and other neoplastic lesions, such as plasmacytoma. Mixed malignant radiolucent and radiopaque lesions also can be observed, such as with osteosarcoma (**Fig. 23**).[120] Purely radiopaque malignant lesions are not found with conditions such as tumoral calcinosis that are considered benign.[121] These malignant lesions can appear in any location in the facial bones. Therefore, clinicians must be thorough in viewing all slices of the CBCT scans to ensure completeness in their evaluation and not miss lesions. Because CBCT scanners can include the entire skull or be partial in view, there is a range of potential findings and diagnoses depending on the FOV window and the type of machine, which affects the potential for liability of practitioners.

Although rarely seen in CBCT studies of dental patients, other types of lesions of concern in the cranial region of the skull are benign and malignant brain tumors. Meningiomas, pituitary adenoma, and acoustic neuromas are examples of benign brain tumors.[122] The pituitary adenoma is an example of a benign brain tumor and it is the growth hormone–secreting type that causes acromegaly seen in an oral and maxillofacial surgery practice due to the associated class III skeletal malocclusion with prognathism and involvement of the sella turcica (**Fig. 24**). Examples of malignant

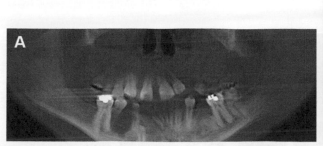
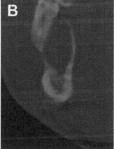

Fig. 15. Right mandibular odontogenic keratocyst (OKC) or Keratocystic odontogenic tumor (KCOT) of Gorlin-Goltz syndrome. (*A*) Panoramic view. (*B*) Sequential oblique sagittal cross sectional images demonstrating close relationship of mandibular canal to the cyst/tumor.

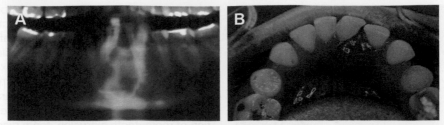

Fig. 16. (*A*) Panoramic view of unicystic ameloblastoma midline mandible. (*B*) Clinical view of bluish raised mucosa of unicystic ameloblatoma.

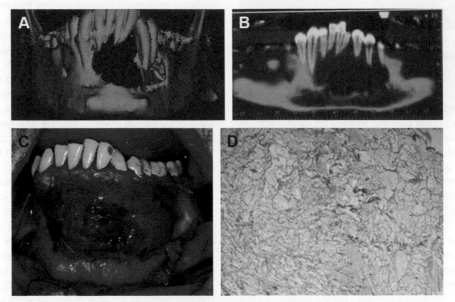

Fig. 17. (*A*) Odontogenic myxoma 3-D CT view of destructive lesion. (*B*) Odontogenic myxoma panoramic CT view of destructive lesion. (*C*) Odontogenic myxoma intraoperative clinical view of destructive lesion. (*D*) Odontogenic myxoma pathology; hematoxylin-eosin stain, low-power view.

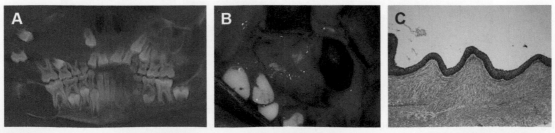

Fig. 18. Odontogenic keratocyst (OKC) or Keratocystic odontogenic tumor (KCOT) of Gorlin-Goltz syndrome. (*A*) Panoramic view. (*B*) Intraoperative clinical view. (*C*) Pathology; hematoxylin-eosin stain, low-power view.

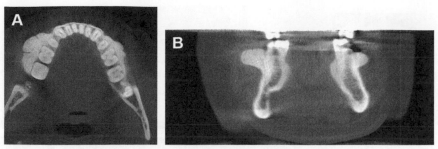

Fig. 19. Exostoses (tori) of bilateral buccal mandible. (*A*) Axial view. (*B*) Coronal view.

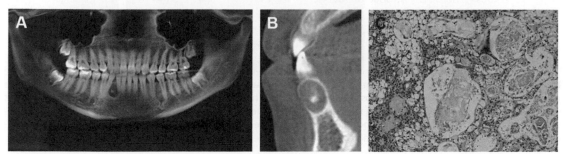

Fig. 20. (*A*) Adenomatoid odontogenic tumor panoramic view lesion between teeth #26 and #27. (*B*) Adenomatoid odontogenic tumor reformatted sagittal view lesion between teeth #26 and #27. (*C*) Adenomatoid odontogenic tumor pathology; hematoxylin-eosin stain, low-power view.

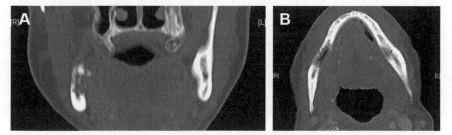

Fig. 21. (*A*) Osteomyelitis of the right mandible coronal view. (*B*) Osteomyelitis of the right mandible axial view.

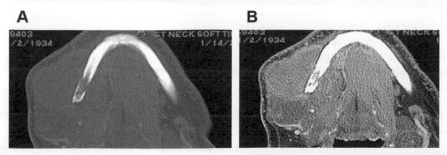

Fig. 22. (*A*) Squamous cell carcinoma invading the right mandible bone window. (*B*) Squamous cell carcinoma invading the right mandible soft tissue window.

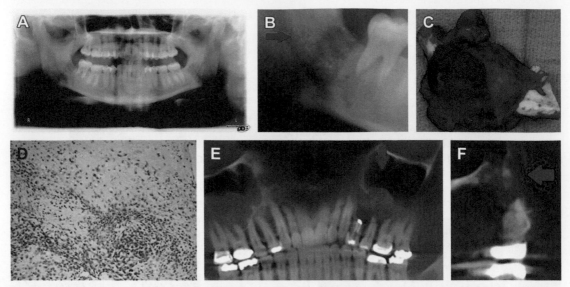

Fig. 23. (*A*) Osteosarcoma of the right mandible panoramic radiograph. (*B*) Osteosarcoma of the right mandible panoramic radiograph close-up. Note loss of cortex distal tooth #31. (*C*) Osteosarcoma of the right mandible gross surgical specimen. (*D*) Osteosarcoma of the right mandible; hematoxylin-eosin stain, low-power view. (*E*) Osteosarcoma of the left maxillary sinus panoramic view. Note mixed radiopaque and radiolucent lesion. (*F*) Osteosarcoma of the left maxilla reformatted sagittal view. Note mixed radiopaque and radiolucent lesion.

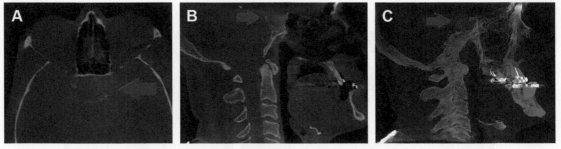

Fig. 24. (*A*) Axial view, pituitary adenoma postsurgical change. (*B*) Sagittal view, pituitary adenoma, postsurgical change. (*C*) Midline sagittal view, pituitary adenoma, postsurgical change.

brain tumors include astrocytomas, gliomas, metastatic cancers, plasmacytoma, multiple myeloma, and skin and scalp tumors, all of which can erode the cranial region of the skull bones and base of skull.[123–128] Within the sinus cavities, various types of benign and malignant lesions can be present. Most common are findings of benign mucous membrane thickening and polyp formation, which includes the classic mucocele (**Fig. 25**).[129,130] Malignant tumors that arise within the confines of the maxillary sinuses are

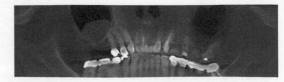

Fig. 25. Maxillary sinus mucocele.

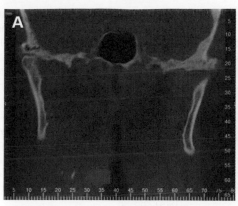
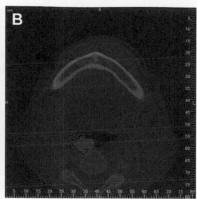

Fig. 26. (*A*) Coronal view, calcified carotid plaque, right neck. (*B*) Axial view, calcified carotid plaque, right neck.

uncommon.[131,132] Evaluation of the frontal, maxillary, and ethmoid sinuses for pathology needs to be complete as well. CBCT, unlike helical CT scanning, is designed for bone imaging and is unable to adequately evaluate the soft tissues, which makes practitioners less liable for isolated lesions of lymph nodes, salivary glands, and associated skin and muscle.

Another entity that can be seen on CBCT scan is calcified carotid plaques seen below the mandible in the region of the bifurcation of the internal and external carotid, which represent calcium deposits within the intima of the carotid vessels.[133,134] Calcified carotid plaques can be observed in the panoramic view,[135] and coronal views as parallel walls (**Fig. 26**A), and axial views as circular (**Fig. 26**B). These lesions must be reported to patients who must be referred to a vascular specialist.

According to sources at a leading oral and maxillofacial surgery liability insurance provider, practitioners are responsible for the interpretation of a CBCT's entire FOV, which in the case of a full FOV can be from vertex to menton.[136–138] There are still open questions as to what is the scope of dental education and extent of diagnostic responsibility.

In conclusion, CBCT has become an important new technology for oral and maxillofacial surgery practitioners and provides improved office-based diagnostic capability and applications for surgical procedures, such as CT guidance through the use of computer-generated drill guides.[139] A thorough knowledge of the basic science of CBCT as well as the ability to interpret the images correctly and thoroughly is essential to current practice.

REFERENCES

1. Scarfe WC, Farman AG, Levin MD, et al. Essentials of maxillofacial cone beam computed tomography. Alpha Omegan 2010;103(2):62–7.
2. Farman AG, Scarfe WC, van Genuchten M. Multi-dimensional imaging: immediate and imminent issues. Compend Contin Educ Dent 2010;31(8): 648–51.
3. Scarfe WC, Farman A, Sukovic P. Clinical applications of cone-beam computed tomography in dental practice. J Can Dent Assoc 2006;72(1): 75–80.
4. Ahmad M, Jenny J, Downie M. Application of cone beam computed tomography in oral and maxillofacial surgery. Aust Dent J 2012;57(Suppl 1):82–94.
5. Chau AC, Fung K. Comparison of radiation dose for implant imaging using conventional spiral tomography, computed tomography, and cone-beam computed tomography. Oral Surg Oral Med Oral Pathol Oral Radiol Endod 2009;107(4):559–65.
6. American Dental Association Council on Scientific Affairs. The use of dental radiographs update and recommendations. J Am Dent Assoc 2006;137: 1304–12.
7. Berdon WE, Slovis TL. Where we are since ALARA and the series of articles on CT dose in children and risk of long-term cancers: what has changed? Pediatr Radiol 2002;32(10):699.
8. Becker A, Chaushu S, Casap-Caspi N. Cone-beam computed tomography and the orthosurgical management of impacted teeth. J Am Dent Assoc 2010;141(Suppl 3):14S–8S.
9. Ghaeminia H, Meijer GJ, Soehardi A, et al. Position of the impacted third molar in relation to the mandibular canal. Diagnostic accuracy of cone beam computed tomography compared with

panoramic radiography. Int J Oral Maxillofac Surg 2009;38(9):964–71.

10. Katheria BC, Kau CH, Tate R, et al. Effectiveness of impacted and supernumerary tooth diagnosis from traditional radiography versus cone beam computed tomography. Pediatr Dent 2010;32(4): 304–9.

11. Palomo L, Palomo JM. Cone beam CT for diagnosis and treatment planning in trauma cases. Dent Clin North Am 2009;53(4):717–27, vi–vii.

12. Naitoh M, Suenaga Y, Kondo S, et al. Assessment of maxillary sinus septa using cone-beam computed tomography:etiological consideration. Clin Implant Dent Relat Res 2009;11(Suppl 1):e52–8.

13. Kuribayashi A, Watanabe H, Imaizumi A, et al. Bifid mandibular canals: cone beam computed tomography evaluation. Dentomaxillofac Radiol 2010; 39(4):235–9.

14. Tyndall DA, Rathore S. Cone-beam CT diagnostic applications: caries, periodontal bone assessment, and endodontic applications. Dent Clin North Am 2008;52(4):825–41, vii.

15. Alkhader M, Kuribayashi A, Ohbayashi N, et al. Usefulness of cone beam computed tomography in temporomandibular joints with soft tissue pathology. Dentomaxillofac Radiol 2010;39(6): 343–8.

16. Barghan S, Merrill R, Tetradis SJ. Cone beam computed tomography imaging in the evaluation of the temporomandibular joint. J Calif Dent Assoc 2010;38(1):33–9.

17. Schneiderman ED, Xu H, Salyer KE. Characterization of the maxillary complex in unilateral cleft lip and palate using cone-beam computed tomography: a preliminary study. J Craniofac Surg 2009; 20(Suppl 2):1699–710.

18. Mah JK, Huang JC, Choo H. Practical applications of cone-beam computed tomography in orthodontics. J Am Dent Assoc 2010;141(Suppl 3):7S–13S.

19. Turpin DL. Clinical guidelines and the use of cone-beam computed tomography. Am J Orthod Dentofacial Orthop 2010;138(1):1–2.

20. Orentlicher G, Goldsmith D, Horowitz A. Applications of 3-dimensional virtual computerized tomography technology in oral and maxillofacial surgery: current therapy. J Oral Maxillofac Surg 2010;68(8): 1933–59.

21. Ilgüy D, Ilgüy M, Fisekcioglu E, et al. Detection of jaw and root fractures using cone beam computed tomography: a case report. Dentomaxillofac Radiol 2009;38(3):169–73.

22. Tetradis S, Anstey P, Graff-Radford S. Cone beam computed tomography in the diagnosis of dental disease. J Calif Dent Assoc 2010;38(1):27–32.

23. Drage NA, Brown JE. Cone beam computed sialography of sialoliths. Dentomaxillofac Radiol 2009;38(5):301–5.

24. Tso HH, Lee JS, Huang JC, et al. Evaluation of the human airway using cone-beam computerized tomography. Oral Surg Oral Med Oral Pathol Oral Radiol Endod 2009;108(5):768–76.

25. Angelopoulos C, Aghaloo T. Imaging technology in implant diagnosis. Dent Clin North Am 2011;55(1): 141–58.

26. Worthington P, Rubenstein J, Hatcher DC. The role of cone-beam computed tomography in the planning and placement of implants. J Am Dent Assoc 2010;141(Suppl 3):19S–24S.

27. Chan HL, Misch K, Wang HL. Dental imaging in implant treatment planning. Implant Dent 2010; 19(4):288–98.

28. Bornstein MM, Scarfe WC, Vaughn VM, et al. Cone beam computed tomography in implant dentistry: a systematic review focusing on guidelines, indications, and radiation dose risks. Int J Oral Maxillofac Implants 2014;29(Suppl):55–77.

29. Vercruyssen M, Cox C, Coucke W, et al. A randomized clinical trial comparing guided implant surgery (bone- or mucosa-supported) with mental navigation or the use of a pilot-drill template. J Clin Periodontol 2014;41(7): 717–23.

30. De Santis D, Canton LC, Cucchi A, et al. Computer-assisted surgery in the lower jaw: double surgical guide for immediately loaded implants in postextractive sites-technical notes and a case report. J Oral Implantol 2010;36(1):61–8.

31. Block MS, Mercante DE, Lirette D, et al. Prospective evaluation of immediate and delayed provisional single tooth restorations. J Oral Maxillofac Surg 2009;67(11 Suppl):89–107.

32. Valente F, Schiroli G, Sbrenna A. Accuracy of computer-aided oral implant surgery: a clinical and radiographic study. Int J Oral Maxillofac Implants 2009;24(2):234–42.

33. Holst S, Blatz MB, Eitner S. Precision for computer-guided implant placement: using 3D planning software and fixed intraoral reference points. J Oral Maxillofac Surg 2007;65(3):393–9.

34. Katsoulis J, Pazera P, Mericske-Stern R. Prosthetically driven, computer-guided implant planning for the edentulous maxilla: a model study. Clin Implant Dent Relat Res 2009;11(3):238–45.

35. Tyndall DA, Price JB, Tetradis S, et al. Position statement of the American Academy of Oral and Maxillofacial Radiology on selection criteria for the use of radiology in dental implantology with emphasis on cone beam computed tomography. Oral Surg Oral Med Oral Pathol Oral Radiol 2012; 113(6):817–26.

36. Meloni SM, De Riu G, Pisano M, et al. Implant treatment software planning and guided flapless surgery with immediate provisional prosthesis delivery in the fully edentulous maxilla. A

retrospective analysis of 15 consecutively treated patients. Eur J Oral Implantol 2010;3(3):245–51.

37. Cogbill TH, Ziegelbein KJ. Computed tomography, magnetic resonance, and ultrasound imaging: basic principles, glossary of terms, and patient safety. Surg Clin North Am 2011;91(1):1–14.

38. Oliva L. Alessandro Vallebona (1899–1987). Radiol Med 1988;76(1–2):127–9.

39. Scarfe WC, Eraso FE, Farman AG. Characteristics of the orthopantomograph OP 100. Dentomaxillofac Radiol 1998;27(1):51–7.

40. Liang H, Frederiksen NL. Focal trough and patient positioning. Dentomaxillofac Radiol 2004;33(2):128–9.

41. Kyrieleis A, Titarenko V, Ibison M, et al. Region-of-interest tomography using filtered backprojection: assessing the practical limits. J Microsc 2011;241(1):69–82.

42. Schultz E, Felix R. Fan-beam computerized tomography systems with rotating and with stationary detector arrays ('third' and 'fourth' generation). Med Prog Technol 1980;7(4):169–81.

43. Beckmann EC. Godfrey newbold hounsfield. Phys Today 2005;58(3):84–5.

44. Oransky I. Sir Godfrey N. Hounsfield. Lancet 2004;364(9439):1032.

45. Beckmann EC. CT scanning the early days. Br J Radiol 2006;79(937):5–8.

46. Shampo MA, Kyle RA. Allan Cormack–codeveloper of computed tomographic scanner. Mayo Clin Proc 1996;71(3):288.

47. Raju TN. The Nobel chronicles. 1979: Allan MacLeod Cormack (b 1924); and Sir Godfrey Newbold Hounsfield (b 1919). Lancet 1999 Nov 6;354(9190):1653.

48. Elke M. One century of diagnostic imaging in medicine. Experientia 1995;51(7):665–80.

49. Rogalla P, Kloeters C, Hein PA. CT technology overview: 64-slice and beyond. Radiol Clin North Am 2009;47(1):1–11.

50. Sittig DF, Ash JS, Ledley RS. The story behind the development of the first whole-body computerized tomography scanner as told by Robert S. Ledley. J Am Med Inform Assoc 2006;13(5):465–9.

51. Goodman LR. The Beatles, the nobel prize, and CT scanning of the chest. Radiol Clin North Am 2010;48(1):1–7.

52. Alexander RE, Gunderman RB. EMI and the first CT scanner. J Am Coll Radiol 2010;7(10):778–81.

53. Petrik V, Apok V, Britton JA, et al. Godfrey Hounsfield and the dawn of computed tomography. Neurosurgery 2006;58(4):780–7 [discussion: 780–7].

54. Schaller S, Flohr T, Steffen P. An efficient Fourier method for 3-D radon inversion in exact cone-beam CT Reconstruction. IEEE Trans Med Imaging 1998;17(2):244–50.

55. Hornich H. A tribute to Johann Radon. IEEE Trans Med Imaging 1986;5(4):169.

56. Katsevich A. Analysis of an exact inversion algorithm for spiral cone-beam CT. Phys Med Biol 2002;47(15):2583–97.

57. Anastasio MA, Pan X, Clarkson E. Comments on the filtered backprojection algorithm, range conditions, and the pseudoinverse solution. IEEE Trans Med Imaging 2001;20(6):539–42.

58. Morvidone M, Nguyen MK, Truong TT, et al. On the v-line radon transform and its imaging applications. Int J Biomed Imaging 2010. pii: 208179. Epub 2010 Jul 13.

59. Kampp TD. The back projection method applied to classical tomography. Med Phys 1986;13(3):329–33.

60. Zhang-O'Connor Y, Fessler JA. Fourier-based forward and back-projectors in iterative fan-beam tomographic image reconstruction. IEEE Trans Med Imaging 2006;25(5):582–9.

61. Wang G, Ye Y, Yu H. Approximate and exact cone-beam reconstruction with standard and non-standard spiral scanning. Phys Med Biol 2007;52(6):R1–13.

62. Kordolaimi SD, Saradeas I, Ploussi A, et al. Introduction of an effective method for the optimization of CT protocols using iterative reconstruction algorithms: comparison with patient data. Am J Roentgenol 2014;203(4):W434–9.

63. Mazin SR, Pelc NJ. Fourier properties of the fan-beam sinogram. Med Phys 2010;37(4):1674–80.

64. Averbuch A, Sedelnikov I, Shkolnisky Y. CT reconstruction from parallel and fan beam projections by a 2D discrete radon transform. IEEE Trans Image Process 2012;21(2):733–41.

65. Pan X, Sidky EY, Vannier M. Why do commercial CT scanners still employ traditional, filtered back-projection for image reconstruction? Inverse Probl 2009;25(12):1230009.

66. Brock RS, Docef A, Murphy MJ. Reconstruction of a cone-beam CT image via forward iterative projection matching. Med Phys 2010;37(12):6212–20.

67. Boas FE, Fleischmann D. Evaluation of two iterative techniques for reducing metal artifacts in computed tomography. Radiology 2011;259:894.

68. Brooks RA. A quantitative theory of the Hounsfield unit and its application to dual energy scanning. J Comput Assist Tomogr 1977;1:487.

69. Hohlweg-Majert B, Metzger MC, Kummer T, et al. Morphometric analysis - cone beam computed tomography to predict bone quality and quantity. J Craniomaxillofac Surg 2011;39:330–4.

70. Reboudi A, Trisi P, Cecchini G. Preoperative evaluation of bone quality and bone density using a novel CT/micro CT based hard normal soft classification system. Int J Oral Maxillofac Implants 2010;25(1):75–85.

71. Turkilmaz I, Ozan O, Yilmaz B, et al. Determination of bone quality of 372 implant recipient sites using hounsfield unit from computerized tomography: a clinical study. Clin Implant Dent Relat Res 2008; 10(4):238–44.

72. Lou SL, Hoogstrate DR, Huang HK. An automated PACS image acquisition and recovery scheme for image integrity based on the DICOM standard. Comput Med Imaging Graph 1997;21(4):209–18.

73. Nagy P. Open source in imaging informatics. J Digit Imaging 2007;20(Suppl 1):1–10.

74. Perandini S, Faccioli N, Zaccarella A, et al. The diagnostic contribution of CT volumetric rendering techniques in routine practice. Indian J Radiol Imaging 2010;20(2):92–7.

75. Kalender WA, Seissler W, Klotz E, et al. Spiral volumetric CT with single-breathhold technique, continuous transport, and continuous scanner rotation. Radiology 1990;176(1):181–3.

76. Kalender WA, Vock P, Polacin A, et al. Spiral-CT: a new technique for volumetric scans. I. Basic principles and methodology. Rontgenpraxis 1990;43(9): 323–30.

77. Soucek M, Vock P, Daepp M, et al. Spiral-CT: a new technique for volumetric scans. II. Potential clinical applications. Rontgenpraxis 1990;43(10):365–75.

78. Gupta R, Cheung AC, Soenke H, et al. Flat-panel volume CT: fundamental principles, technology, and applications. Radiographics 2008; 28:2009–22.

79. Baba R, Ueda K, Okabe M. Using a flat-panel detector in high resolution cone beam CT for dental imaging. Dentomaxillofac Radiol 2004; 33(5):285–90.

80. Draenert FG, Coppenrath E, Herzog P, et al. Beam hardening artefacts occur in dental implant scans with the NewTom cone beam CT but not with the dental 4-row multidetector CT. Dentomaxillofac Radiol 2007;36(4):198–203.

81. Brenner DJ, Hall EJ. Computed tomography–an increasing source of radiation exposure. N Engl J Med 2007;357(22):2277–84.

82. Berrington de González A, Mahesh M, Kim KP, et al. Projected cancer risks from computed tomographic scans performed in the United States in 2007. Arch Intern Med 2009;169(22):2071–7.

83. Pauwels R, Cockmartin L, Ivanauskaité D, et al, SEDENTEXCT Project Consortium. Estimating cancer risk from dental cone-beam CT exposures based on skin dosimetry. Phys Med Biol 2014; 59(14):3877–91.

84. Shuryak I, Sachs RK, Brenner DJ. A new view of radiation induced cancer. Radiat Prot Dosimetry 2011;143(2-4):358–64.

85. Brenner DJ. Slowing the increase in the population dose resulting from CT scans. Radiat Res 2010; 174(6):809–15. Epub 2010 Aug 23.

86. Lee CY, Koval TM, Suzuki JB. Low dose radiation risks of CT and CBCT: reducing the fear and controversy. J Oral Implantol 2014. [Epub ahead of print].

87. Brenner D, Elliston C, Hall E, et al. Estimated risks of radiation-induced fatal cancer from pediatric CT. AJR Am J Roentgenol 2001;176(2):289–96.

88. Ludlow JB, Davies-Ludlow LE, White SC. Patient risk related to common dental radiographic examination examinations: the impact of 2007 International Commission on Radiological Protection recommendations regarding dose calculation. J Am Dent Assoc 2008;139:1237–43.

89. National Council on Radiation Protection and Measurements. Ionizing radiation exposure of the population of the United States. Bethesda (MD): National Council on Radiation Protection and Measurements; 2006. NCRP Report No. 160.

90. Roberts JA, Drage NA, Davies J, et al. Effective dose from cone beam CT examinations in dentistry. Br J Radiol 2009;82:35–40.

91. De Vos W, Casselman J, Swennen GR. Cone-beam computerized tomography (CBCT) imaging of the oral and maxillofacial region: a systematic review of the literature. Int J Oral Maxillofac Surg 2009; 38(6):609–25.

92. Mettler FA, Huda W, Yoshizumi TT, et al. Effective doses in radiology and diagnostic nuclear medicine: a catalog. Radiology 2008;248(1):254–63.

93. Brenner DJ, Elliston CD. Estimated radiation risks potentially associated with full-body CT screening. Radiology 2004;232(3):735–8.

94. Magnusson B, Borrman H. The paradental cyst a clinicopathologic study of 26 cases. Swed Dent J 1995;19(1-2):1–7.

95. Weber AL. Imaging of cysts and odontogenic tumors of the jaw. Definition and classification. Radiol Clin North Am 1993;31(1):101–20.

96. Baykul T, Saglam AA, Aydin U, et al. Incidence of cystic changes in radiographically normal impacted lower third molar follicles. Oral Surg Oral Med Oral Pathol Oral Radiol Endod 2005; 99(5):542–5.

97. Simon JH, Enciso R, Malfaz JM, et al. Differential diagnosis of large periapical lesions using cone-beam computed tomography measurements and biopsy. J Endod 2006;32(9):833–7.

98. Cassatly MG, Greenberg AM, Kopp WK. Bilateral giant cell granulomata of the mandible: report of case. J Am Dent Assoc 1988;117(6):731–3.

99. Cohen MA, Hertzanu Y. Radiologic features, including those seen with computed tomography, of central giant cell granuloma of the jaws. Oral Surg Oral Med Oral Pathol 1988; 65(2):255–61.

100. DeTomasi D, Hann JR. Traumatic bone cyst: report of case. J Am Dent Assoc 1985;111(1):56–7.

101. Sun ZJ, Zhao YF, Yang RL, et al. Aneurysmal bone cysts of the jaws: analysis of 17 cases. J Oral Maxillofac Surg 2010;68(9):2122–8.

102. Marks R, Block M, Sanusi ID, et al. Unicytic ameloblastoma. Int J Oral Surg 1983;12:186–9.

103. Singer SR, Mupparapu M, Philipone E. Cone-beam computed tomography findings in a case of plexiform ameloblastoma. Quintessence Int 2009;40: 627.

104. Araki M, Kameodka S, Matsumato N, et al. Usefulness of cone-beam computed tomography for odontogenic myxoma. Dentomaxillofac Radiol 2007;36:423.

105. Madras J, Lapointe H. Keratocystic odontogenic tumor: reclassification of the odontogenic keratocyst from cyst to tumour. J Can Dent Assoc 2008; 74:165.

106. Kaffe I, Ardekian L, Taicher S, et al. Radiologic features of central giant cell granuloma of the jaws. Oral Surg Oral Med Oral Pathol Radiol Endod 1996;81(6):720–6.

107. Kamel SG, Kau CH, Wong ME, et al. The role of Cone beam CT in the evaluation and management of a family with Gardner's syndrome. J Craniomaxillofac Surg 2009;37(8):461–8.

108. Manganaro AM, Millett GV. Periapical cemental dysplasia. Gen Dent 1996;44(4):336–9.

109. Ackermann GL, Altini M. The cementomas–a clinicopathological re-appraisal. J Dent Assoc S Afr 1992;47(5):187–94.

110. Abrahams JJ, Berger SB. Inflammatory disease of the jaw: appearance on reformatted CT scans. AJR Am J Roentgenol 1998;170(4):1085–91.

111. Boeddinghaus R, Whyte A. Current concepts in maxillofacial imaging. Eur J Radiol 2008;66(3): 396–418.

112. Su L, Weathers DR, Waldron CA. Distinguished features of focal cemento-osseous dysplasia and cemento-ossifying fibroma II. A clinical and radiologic spectrum of 316 cases. Oral Surg Oral Med Oral Pathol Oral Radiol Endod 1997;84:540–9.

113. Ribeiro AC, Carlos R, Díaz KP. Bilateral central ossifying fibroma affecting the mandible report of an uncommon case and critical review of the literature. Oral Surg Oral Med Oral Pathol Oral Radiol Endod 2011;111(2):e21–6.

114. Cavalcanti MG, Ruprecht A, Vannier MW. Evaluation of an ossifying fibroma using three-dimensional computed tomography. Dentomaxillofac Radiol 2001;30(6):342–5.

115. Philipsen HP, Reichart PA, Siar CH, et al. An updated clinical and epidemiological profile of the adenomatoid odontogenic tumour: a collaborative retrospective study. J Oral Pathol Med 2007; 36(7):383–93.

116. Cross JJ, Pilkington RJ, Antoun NM, et al. Value of computed tomography and magnetic resonance imaging in the treatment of a calcifying epithelial odontogenic (Pindborg) tumour. Br J Oral Maxillofac Surg 2000;38(2):154–7.

117. Ida M, Tetsumura A, Kurabayashi T, et al. Periosteal new bone formation in the jaws. A computed tomographic study. Dentomaxillofac Radiol 1997;26(3): 169–76.

118. Hariya Y, Yuasa K, Nakayama E, et al. Value of computed tomography findings in differentiating between intraosseous malignant tumors and osteomyelitis of the mandible affecting the masticator space. Oral Surg Oral Med Oral Pathol Oral Radiol Endod 2003;95(4):503–9.

119. Hendrikx AW, Maal T, Dieleman F, et al. Cone beam CT in the assessment of mandibular invasion by oral squamous cell carcinoma: results of the preliminary study. Int J Oral Maxillofac Surg 2010; 39(5):436–9.

120. Closmann JJ, Schmidt BL. The use of cone beam computed tomography as an aid in evaluating and treatment planning for mandibular cancer. J Oral Maxillofac Surg 2007;65(4):766–71.

121. Gal G, Metzker A, Garlick J, et al. Head and neck manifestations of tumoral calcinosis. Oral Surg Oral Med Oral Pathol 1994;77(2):158–66.

122. Black PM. Benign brain tumors. Meningiomas, pituitary tumors, and acoustic neuromas. Neurol Clin 1995;13(4):927–52.

123. Emsen IM. A great Marjolin's ulcer of the scalp invading outer calvarial bone and its different treatment with support of Medpor. J Craniofac Surg 2008;19(4):1026–9.

124. Ertas U, Yalcin E, Erdogan F. Invasive ductal carcinoma with multiple metastases to facial and cranial bones: a case report. Eur J Dent 2010;4(3):334–7.

125. Gheyi V, Hui FK, Doppenberg EM, et al. Broaddus glioblastoma multiforme causing calvarial destruction: an unusual manifestation revisited. AJNR Am J Neuroradiol 2004;25(9):1533–7.

126. Schick U, Bleyen J, Bani A, et al. Management of meningiomas en plaque of the sphenoid wing. J Neurosurg 2006;104(2):208–14.

127. Akutsu H, Sugita K, Sonobe M, et al. Parasagittal meningioma en plaque with extracranial extension presenting diffuse massive hyperostosis of the skull. Surg Neurol 2004;61(2):165–9 [discussion: 169].

128. Singh AD, Chacko AG, Chacko G, et al. Plasma cell tumors of the skull. Surg Neurol 2005;64(5): 434–8 [discussion: 438–9].

129. Arrué P, Kany MT, Serrano E, et al. Mucoceles of the paranasal sinuses: uncommon location. J Laryngol Otol 1998;112(9):840–4.

130. Marks SC, Latoni JD, Mathog RH. Mucoceles of the maxillary sinus. Otolaryngol Head Neck Surg 1997; 117(1):18–21.

131. da Cruz Perez DE, Pires FR, Lopes MA, et al. Adenoid cystic carcinoma and mucoepidermoid

carcinoma of the maxillary sinus: report of a 44-year experience of 25 cases from a single institution. J Oral Maxillofac Surg 2006;64(11):1592–7.

132. Gregoire C, Adler D, Madey S, et al. Basosquamous carcinoma involving the anterior skull base: a neglected tumor treated using intraoperative navigation as a guide to achieve safe resection margins. J Oral Maxillofac Surg 2011;69(1): 230–6.

133. Uwatoko T, Toyoda K, Inoue T, et al. Carotid artery calcification on multislice detector-row computed tomography. Cerebrovasc Dis 2007;24(1):20–6.

134. Wintermark M, Jawadi SS, Rapp JH, et al. High-resolution CT imaging of carotid artery atherosclerotic plaques. AJNR Am J Neuroradiol 2008;29(5): 875–82.

135. Almog DM, Illig KA, Carter LC, et al. Diagnosis of non-dental conditions. Carotid artery calcifications on panoramic radiographs identify patients at risk for stroke. N Y State Dent J 2004;70(8):20–5.

136. Curley A, Hatcher DC. Cone beam CT–anatomic assessment and legal issues: the new standards of care. J Calif Dent Assoc 2009;37(9): 653–62.

137. Macdonald-Jankowski DS, Orpe EC. Some current legal issues that may affect oral and maxillofacial radiology. Part 2: digital monitors and cone-beam computed tomography. J Can Dent Assoc 2007; 73(6):507–11.

138. Plunkett L. A diagnostic dilemma. N Y State Dent J 2010;76(6):6–7.

139. Greenberg A. Basics of Cone-Beam CT and CT Guided Dental Implant Surgery Selected Readings in Oral and Maxillofacial Surgery 2011; 19(5):1–48.

Simple Bone Augmentation for Alveolar Ridge Defects

Christopher J. Haggerty, DDS, MD[a,b,*],
Christopher T. Vogel, DDS[b], G. Rawleigh Fisher, DDS, MD[c]

KEYWORDS

- Osteoconductive • Osteoinductive • Bone grafting • Alveolar defect • Block graft augmentation
- Ramus graft • Chin graft • Socket preservation graft

KEY POINTS

- Alveolar augmentation is frequently required to restore volume lost as a result of disuse atrophy (acquired and congenital), dentoalveolar trauma, infection, periodontal disease, traumatic extractions, and previous failed implant insertion.
- Practitioners are required to have a basic understanding of grafting principles, bone physiology, autogenous graft harvest techniques, and modern grafting materials to reliably and predictably restore lost alveolar volume.
- Numerous grafting materials are available for alveolar reconstruction and include autografts, allografts, xenografts, synthetic grafts, and osteoinductive agents.
- Numerous grafting options are available for in-office use, including socket preservation grafting, particulate onlay grafting, block onlay grafting, ridge split, interpositional osteotomy, distraction osteogenesis, and guided barrier regeneration.
- As bone sources continue to evolve, the previous "gold standard" will continue to shift toward non-autogenous sources and shorter treatment times.

INTRODUCTION

The global dental implant market was valued at approximately $6.8 billion in 2011 and is estimated to grow at a compound annual growth rate of 9% per year between 2011 and 2016.[1] In 2013, an estimated 1,260,000 dental implant procedures were performed in the United States, and this number is expected to double within the next 7 years.[2] The US dental implant market is currently valued at approximately $900 million and is expected to grow at a rate of 9% per year between 2011 and 2021.[2,3] As the perceived profitability of dental implants increases, so does the number of "implant surgeons" within the market place. In 2006, the American Academy of Implant Dentistry estimated

that of the number of dentists placing dental implants, 56% were general dentists.[2] As the number of general practitioners placing dental implants increases, the complexity of implant and grafting procedures performed by the oral and maxillofacial surgeon will continue to increase, as the simpler cases are "cherry picked" by our general dentistry colleagues. It is auspicious that oral and maxillofacial surgeons' advanced knowledge of oral anatomy and grafting principles will enable continued success and advancements in dental implants and alveolar bone grafting.

Many patients who desire dental implant placement present with significant alveolar bone loss as a result of disuse atrophy (acquired and congenital), dentoalveolar trauma, infection, periodontal

[a] Private Practice, Lakewood Oral and Maxillofacial Surgery Specialists, Lee's Summit, MO, USA; [b] Department of Oral and Maxillofacial Surgery, University of Missouri-Kansas City, Kansas City, MO, USA; [c] Private Practice, Lake Charles Oral and Facial Surgery, Lake Charles, LA, USA
* Corresponding author. Lakewood Oral and Maxillofacial Surgery Specialists, Lee's Summit, MO, USA.
E-mail address: christopherhaggerty@hotmail.com

Oral Maxillofacial Surg Clin N Am 27 (2015) 203–226
http://dx.doi.org/10.1016/j.coms.2015.01.011
1042-3699/15/$ – see front matter © 2015 Elsevier Inc. All rights reserved.

disease, traumatic extractions, and previous failed implant insertion.[4] Before dental implant placement, alveolar ridge augmentation procedures are frequently required to correct reverse maxillomandibular relationships, to correct vertical distance discrepancies between the jaws, to re-create ideal interarch occlusal relationships,[5,6] and to add sufficient bone volume to allow for restoration-driven implant placement. Fortunately, although the harvest of extra-oral bone is typically required to reconstruct large bone defects, most alveolar ridge defects are amendable to reconstruction with alloplastic bone, osteoinductive agents, or the harvest of bone from intraoral sites.[7]

Numerous grafting options are available for alveolar reconstruction and include autografts, allografts, xenografts, synthetic grafts, and osteoinductive agents. Most practitioners realize the advantages and disadvantages of the available grafting materials and select various grafting options based on the location, size, and nature of the site to be augmented. For argument's sake, the ideal grafting material would exhibit a combination of osteogenic, osteoconductive, and osteoinductive properties. It would possess high rates of incorporation with inconsequential resorption and minimal morbidity, provide reliable and proven long-term success rates, and be cost-effective.[4,7–10] In addition, the ideal graft material would allow for the sufficient bulk of bone to be regenerated that would allow for recontouring according to the recipient site and permit the placement of dental implants within the healed graft with a high success rate.[8]

The selection of a grafting procedure is based on the amount of bone missing from the recipient site, the restorative-driven treatment plan (number and location of desired dental implants), the availability of adjacent intraoral donor sites, the patient's willingness to accept complications, and the implant-to-crown time frame (1-stage vs 2-stage procedures). Autogenous grafts have often been referred to as the "gold standard" because they possess osteogenic, osteoconductive, and osteoinductive properties. However, autogenous grafts are often unpredictable, involve a second surgical site, have a higher morbidity than nonautogenous grafts, increased operating time, increased cost, and thus, are frequently unacceptable to the patient because of the abovementioned issues. When possible, intraoral bone harvesting is preferred to extraoral (cranium, hip, tibia) harvesting to eliminate the need for endotracheal anesthesia, gait disturbances, prolonged hospitalizations, and thus, added patient recovery and expense. Bone from a bottle (alloplastic, xenograft, and synthetic bone) eliminates the potential complications associated with the donor site, but typically lacks osteoinductive characteristics and the ability to transfer osteoprogenitor cells to the recipient site. Agents such as bone morphogenic proteins (BMP) possess osteoinductive properties without involving a second surgical site, but are often cost prohibitive and, depending on the site, are often used as an off-label application.

GRAFTING NOMENCLATURE
Autografts

Autografts are grafts harvested from the same individual (genetic match). They are typically considered the "gold standard" because autogenous grafts encompass all 3 mechanisms of bone healing (osteogenesis, osteoconduction, and osteoinduction).[11,12] Advantages of autogenous grafts include its nonimmunogenic characteristics, osteogenic potential, affordability, and the ability to acquire cancellous, cortical, or combination grafts depending on the requirements of the recipient site. Disadvantages of autografts include donor site morbidity, prolonged operating times, and lower patient acceptance rates.[13]

Allografts

Allografts are grafts harvested from the same species, but are genetically different. They may be fresh, frozen, freeze-dried (lyophilized), mineralized, or demineralized. Most allografts are osteoconductive, although some possess osteoinductive properties as well. Advantages of allografts include a lack of donor site morbidity, shortened operating times, and numerous configurations of grafting mediums. Disadvantages of allografts include the inability to transplant osteoprogenitor cells, patient unwillingness to have cadaveric bone grafts due to the potential for disease transfer, and the fact that most allografts lack considerable osteoinductive capability.[14]

Xenografts

Xenografts are grafts that are derived from the inorganic portion of bone from a different species (ie, bovine and porcine). Xenografts share many of the advantages of allografts, but debate exists concerning their efficacy compared with allografts. Compared with allografts, xenografts are reported to have increased connective tissue ingrowth, delayed vascularization, and slower rates of resorption.[15,16]

Alloplastic (Synthetic) Grafts

Alloplastic (synthetic) grafts are grafts derived from nonbiologic materials, such as hydroxyapatite, calcium sulfate, and bioactive glass. Relatively few indications exist for the use of synthetic bone substitutes before implant reconstruction because of nonoptimal physiologic bone turnover and implant osseointegration.[17,18]

BONE GRAFT PHYSIOLOGY

Generation of bone occurs through 3 possible mechanisms: osteogenesis, osteoconduction, and osteoinduction. *Osteogenesis* occurs when surviving osteoprogenitor cells within a grafted material differentiate into osteoblasts and form new bone within the recipient site. Currently, autogenous grafts represent the only available graft with osteogenic capability. *Osteoconduction* occurs when grafted material functions as a scaffold for the ingrowth of vascular tissue and mesenchymal cells from the recipient site. Bone apposition occurs within the graft site, and the grafted material is eventually resorbed and replaced with viable bone. Examples of osteoconductive grafts include allografts, xenografts, and synthetic grafts. *Osteoinduction* involves new bone formation through the recruitment and stimulation of recipient site osteoprogenitor cells using bone growth factors transplanted within the grafted material.[19] Examples of osteoinductive materials include rhBMP-2 Infuse (Medtronic, Memphis, TN, USA)[20] and BMP potentially released during the demineralization process of banked bone.

CORTICAL VERSUS PARTICULATE (CANCELLOUS) BONE

Sources of the cortical bone used for alveolar ridge augmentation include autogenous symphysis,

ramus, and allograft blocks. Cortical bone heals by a process referred to as creeping substitution, whereby the graft undergoes resorption with simultaneous replacement with viable bone.[11] Revascularization of the cortical graft begins at the periphery of the block graft and slowly proceeds toward the interior of the graft. The entire revascularization process takes months and is often incomplete as areas of necrotic bone persist within the graft indefinitely, sealed off from the viable, vascularized regions of the graft.[21] The resorption rates of cortical grafts are highly variable within the literature (0%–50%)[7,10] with most cortical graft resorption occurring at the periphery of the graft.[22] Advantages of mandibular cortical grafts include a high concentration of BMPs,[23] a dense segment of bone that is amendable to rigid fixation to the recipient site, initial primary graft stability, and the development of cortical D-1 to cortical D-2 bone within the recipient site.[24] Disadvantages of cortical grafts include reduced osteogenic activity, high failure rates with early exposure, the need to contour the block graft to passively fit the recipient site, slow rates of revascularization, and incomplete bone replacement.[6,25]

Sources of particulate bone include cancellous bone from the maxillary tuberosity, trephine harvests taken from numerous intraoral sites, bone scrapings from the ramus and tuberosity, and allograft, xenoplastic, and alloplastic sources (**Fig. 1**). Particulate autografts contain high concentrations of osteocompetent cells derived from the trabecular endosteum and cellular marrow, which are hypothesized to initially survive through plasmatic circulation.[19] Particulate grafts heal via a

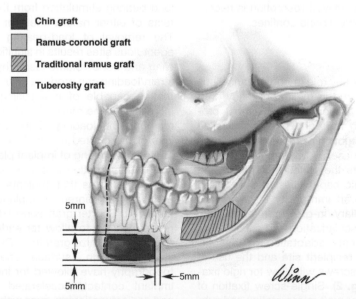

■ Chin graft

▨ Ramus-coronoid graft

▨ Traditional ramus graft

▨ Tuberosity graft

5mm

5mm

5mm

Winn

Fig. 1. Common sources of autogenous bone.

process referred to as rapid incorporation. Rapid incorporation involves the rapid revascularization of the grafted bone because the large trabecular spaces within the cancellous graft allow for the unobstructed invasion of vascular tissue and the diffusion of nutrients within the grafted particulate bone. Rapid incorporation is thought to promote osteoprogenitor cell survival, conveying increased osteogenesis compared with cortical grafts.[25] Compared with their cortical counterparts, cancellous grafts possess more osteogenic activity, allow for more rapid and complete revascularization, and are ultimately completely replaced with new bone within weeks to months. Disadvantages of particulate grafts include the inability to rigidly fixate the grafted material, the frequent need for membranes or titanium mesh, the lack of initial mechanical stability, and the lack of immediate structural support.

DEMINERALIZED VERSUS MINERALIZED

Demineralized bone is obtained after acid dissolution removes the mineral phase of bone, exposing its organic substructure and osteoinductive growth factors (BMPs). Mineralized bone, although not osteoinductive, functions as a more ideal scaffold for the migration of mesenchymal cells into the graft site compared with demineralized bone.[26,27] Because of the rapid incorporation of mineralized allografts within 5 wall socket defects, mineralized allogenic grafts typically allow for faster implant placement and osseointegration compared with demineralized grafts.[16] Demineralized grafts are frequently used for sinus and onlay augmentation procedures wherein delayed resorption is necessary because of nonideal bone confines.

GRAFT FIXATION

Graft fixation plays a key role in corticocancellous block graft survival and in minimizing early graft volume loss. Graft fixation exerts its most profound effects during the early phase of healing by minimizing micromotion of the graft during the revascularization phase.[28] Micromotion of the grafted area disrupts the vascular ingrowth and slows the osteogenic capabilities of the grafted area.[24] Complete graft immobility is paramount to successful capillary in-growth, inosculation, and thus, graft revascularization and survival. For cortical grafts, intimate adaptation of the harvested bone to the recipient site and the use of at least 2 positional screws will allow for rigid fixation of the graft (**Fig. 2**). Single-screw fixation of block grafts allows for graft microrotation and subsequent capillary shearing.[29] Particulate grafts

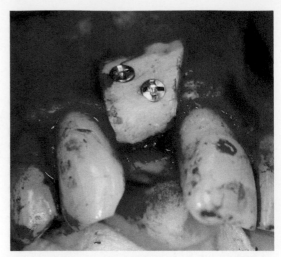

Fig. 2. Symphysis block graft used to augment the horizontal and vertical dimensions of an anterior maxillary alveolus defect. Graft stability and antirotation of the graft is achieved through rigid fixation with 2 positional screws.

may be fixated using membranes to maintain graft position and dimensions, by graft site selection, by using products that come in a moldable paste, and by using tissue adhesives such as fibrin sealants to turn a particulate graft into a more rigid and moldable graft.

GRAFT LOADING

Alveolar bone requires stimulation to maintain its dimensions. Functional levels of bone mass will only be maintained under the effects of continued load-bearing stimulation from the masticatory effects of either natural teeth or loaded implants. The removal of load-bearing stimulation from edentulous sites results in significant bone remodeling and bone volume loss. Physiologic levels of strain/loading can produce an osteogenic stimulus that is capable of maintaining bone level and increasing bone mass.[30,31] Bone grafting without restoring the loading of the bone will result in loss of the grafted material via disuse atrophy.[32] The optimal timing of implant placement following ridge augmentation is controversial in the literature. Most agree that implants should be placed once a high degree of implant stability can be achieved. Shorter graft consolidation periods are recommended to allow for earlier loading of implants to minimize graft loss. Recent advances in implant design, surface characteristics, and topography have allowed for increased bone-to-implant contact, accelerated osseointegration, and earlier functioning, even with the use of shorter length implants. Most grafted extraction sockets can have dental implants placed within 3 to 6 months depending on the radiographic findings. Cortiocancellous block grafts usually require at least 6 months for adequate healing and graft consolidation for implant placement.

PREOPERATIVE PLANNING

Before any augmentation procedure, patients are forewarned about the potential for iatrogenic injury to adjacent teeth, the maxillary sinus, and the inferior alveolar nerve, and that graft success and future implant placement are not guaranteed. Preoperative films are crucial to identify the exact location of key structures (tooth roots, the mandibular canal, the mental foramen, the maxillary sinus) and to define the anatomy of the recipient site, and, with autogenous grafting, the anatomy of the donor site. Cone beam computed tomography (CBCT) or medical grade scans are preferred because of the ability to evaluate the patient's anatomy in 3 dimensions and to precisely measure the location of key structures and of the amount of bone both lateral and superior to key structures. Orthopantomograms may also be used; however, additional periapical films are recommended to adjust for the 20% to 25% magnification error associated with orthopantomogram films. Articulated dental models (stone or digital scanner–generated) will aid in an understanding of the anatomy of the edentulous site and of the amount of augmentation required to appropriately reconstruct alveolar defects. Integration of CBCT scans, intraoral digital scanner data and dental implant planning software, which can include computer-generated surgical guide fabrication, will allow for restoration-driven treatment planning of alveolar augmentation and future dental implant placement (**Table 1**).

SOCKET PRESERVATION GRAFTING

Alveolar ridge preservation is superior to regeneration. Following extractions, a reduction in the alveolar osseous dimension is inevitable. Most of the osseus loss occurs within the first few months after extraction and occurs in a predictable paradigm. Bone loss is more pronounced from the buccal surface compared with the lingual/palatal surface, from the anterior to the posterior aspects of the jaws, from the horizontal to the vertical dimensions of the alveolus, and from the maxilla compared with the mandible.[33–39] Increased trauma at the time of extraction has also been shown to increase the amount of associated bone loss. The resultant byproduct of unassisted extraction site healing is a shorter and narrower alveolar ridge with a lingually positioned crest,

often precluding the placement of dental implants without alveolar augmentation procedures or without ideal angulations for stock abutments.

The morphology of the extraction site affects the predictability of the grafting procedure. The ideal recipient site is a 5-wall defect, thus preserving all bony walls (mesial, distal, lingual/palatal, buccal, and apical). Minimal flap reflection, atraumatic extractions, and preservation of interseptal bone also add to the overall maintenance of osseus volume. Socket preservation grafting does not inhibit alveolar resorption, but aids in maintaining the osseus dimension of the extraction site by limiting the progression of the resorptive process by providing a matrix for osseus healing. Socket preservation grafting allows the surgeon the ability to predictably and precisely minimize the amount of alveolar bone loss that is known to occur after tooth extraction.[40]

Socket Preservation Grafting Procedure

Teeth are extracted atraumatically with preservation of maximum bone (**Fig. 3**A–C) with the use of dental elevators, piezoelectric devices, periotomes, osteotomes, and hand pieces with copious irrigation to section multirooted teeth. Preservation of the buccal plate is paramount to minimize the development of a lingual to buccal sloped ridge. Following extraction, any granulation and abscessed tissue is removed, and the site is judiciously curetted and irrigated. Particulate graft material is hydrated (see **Fig. 3**D) and deposited within the extraction site (see **Fig. 3**E–G). The authors prefer to use mineralized cadaveric bone for socket preservation procedures because of its rapid incorporation, ideal handling characteristics, and shorter overall treatment times compared with demineralized grafts, xenografts, and synthetic grafts. The graft is condensed within the extraction site (see **Fig. 3**H) and covered with either resorbable membranes, local tissue advancements, or both. For maxillary extraction sites, where there is little to no moveable tissue, a collagen membrane or cut collaplug (see **Fig. 3**I) is used to cover the graft material. For mandibular extraction sites or for multiple, adjacent extractions, local advancement flaps with periosteal releasing incisions are typically used, with or without a collagen membrane, depending on the size of the defect and the ability to obtain a tension-free closure. Interrupted or continuous 4-0 chromic sutures are used to provide membrane integrity and tissue closure (see **Fig. 3**I–V). Oral tissue adhesives (PeriAcryl; Glustitch, Delta, BC, Canada) may be used as an adjunct for large maxillary molar extraction sites.

Table 1
Summary chart for alveolar augmentation

Type of Graft	Indications	Type of Ridge Augmentation	Potential Vertical Gain	Potential Horizontal Gain	Maximum Available	Time to Implant Placement	Comments
Socket preservation	Preservation of alveolar volume following extraction	Preventative	Preventative	Preventative	Dependent on socket morphology	See comments	Time until implant placement depends on the material used for preservation: mineralized graft 3–4 mo, demineralized graft 4–5 mo, and bovine graft 5–8 mo
Particulate onlay	Horizontal ridge augmentation	Horizontal	None	1–4 mm	N/A	3–4 mo	Best used for narrow ridges with adequate height and "J"-shaped (3–4 wall bony defects) defects; the anterior maxilla, saddle depressions, and exposed buccal implant threads
Ramus onlay	Horizontal, vertical, or combined ridge augmentation	Horizontal, vertical	3–4 mm	3–4 mm	Traditional ramus 30 × 13 × 2.5 mm	4–6 mo	Purely cortical graft. Highest yield of intraoral bone compared with all other intraoral sources
Symphysis onlay	Horizontal, vertical, or combined ridge augmentation	Horizontal, vertical	4–6 mm	4–6 mm	21 × 10 × 7 mm	4–6 mo	Combined corticocancellous graft with greater depth than ramus graft
Ridge split	Increasing alveolar ridge width	Horizontal	None	2–5 mm (average 3 mm)	N/A	Immediate vs 3–4 mo	Requires preoperative ridge width of 4 mm. Implants may be placed at the time of ridge split

Technique	Indications	Direction			Limiting factor	Timing	Comments
Interpositional graft	Vertical gain in excess of 4 mm	Vertical	5 mm anterior maxilla, 8 mm posterior mandible	None	Limited by lingual soft tissue pedicle	Immediate vs 3–4 mo	Existing soft tissue envelope limits vertical augmentation height. Indicated in instances where onlay grafting is contraindicated (sites requiring 4 mm or more of vertical augmentation)
Distraction osteogenesis	Need for both hard and soft tissue augmentation	Vertical	3–20 mm	None	N/A	3–4 mo after graft consolidation	Often requires overdistraction to achieve desired results. Additional grafting procedures (onlay grafting) are typically required. Can be difficult to control vector of distraction
Guided barrier regeneration	Horizontal, vertical, or combined ridge augmentation	Horizontal, vertical	2–4 mm	3–6 mm	N/A	9–12 mo	Membranes facilitate bone formation through space maintenance and by minimizing the ingrowth of connective tissues and epithelial cells. Early premature exposure often leads to complete graft loss. Late premature exposure often leads to partial graft loss with excellent oral hygiene

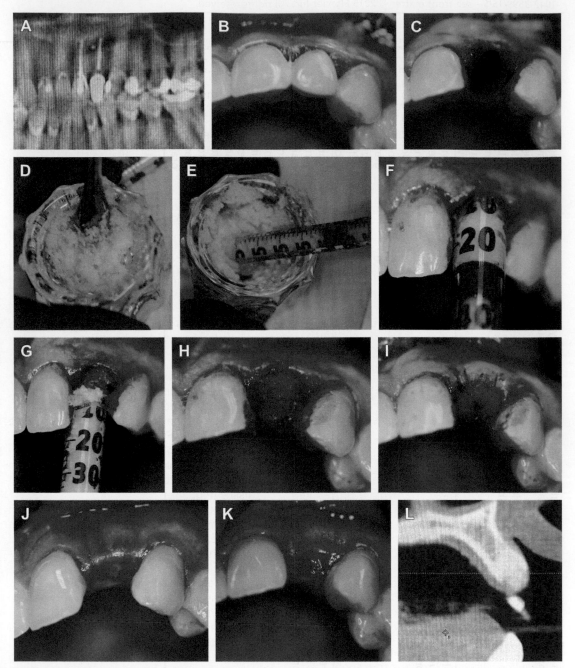

Fig. 3. (*A*) Preoperative orthopantomogram demonstrating an apical abscess and internal resorption of tooth number 10. (*B*) Preoperative view of failing tooth number 10. (*C*) Tooth number 10 extracted atraumatically with preservation of the buccal plate and minimal flap elevation. (*D, E*). Hydration of mineralized cadaveric bone and placement into a Tb syringe carrier. (*F, G*) Mineralized cadaveric bone is placed within the extraction site using a Tb syringe as a carrier. (*H*) The graft is condensed within the extraction site. (*I*) A section of collaplug is placed over the extraction/graft site and secured in place with figure-of-eight 4-0 chromic sutures. (*J*) Site after 3 weeks of healing. (*K*) Site after 6 weeks of healing. (*L*) Fourteen-week sagittal CBCT scan shows excellent graft consolidation and retention. (*M*) Virtual surgical treatment planning of implant number 10 in grafted site. (*N*) Occlusal view of virtual implant placement designed for a screw-retained final prosthesis. (*O*) Site before implant placement at 16 weeks. (*P*) Placement of surgical guide. (*Q, R*) Drill sleeves are used to sequentially enlarge the implant osteotomy. (*S, T*) Implant is placed via flapless technique. (*U, V*) Final placement of implant correlates with preoperative workup.

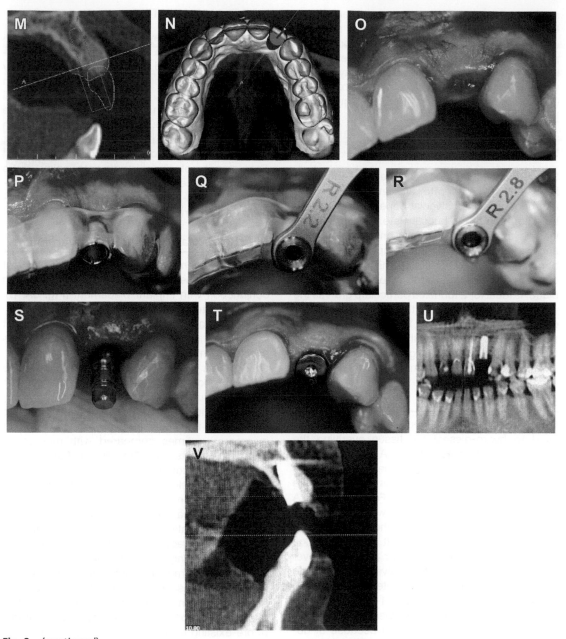

Fig. 3. (*continued*)

ONLAY GRAFTING

Onlay grafting is performed when augmentation is required in either a vertical, a horizontal, or combined dimension to allow for sufficient implant length, width, and location. Onlay grafting may be categorized as either particulate or block/corticocancellous in nature. Ridge morphology dictates the type of onlay graft utilized. Three-wall and four-wall bony defects, saddle depressions, and areas of deficient buccal bone with an inferior

stop are typically amendable to onlay particulate grafting. Two-wall bony defects respond best to block onlay grafting procedures.

PARTICULATE ONLAY GRAFTS

Particulate graft sources include any combination of autogenous, alloplastic, xenoplastic, and synthetic bone, may be prepackaged within a bone putty (Regenaform; Exactech, Gainesville, FL, USA), mixed with a tissue adhesive to provide support and form (Tisseel; Baxter, Deerfield, IL, USA), or combined with osteoinductive materials (rhBMP-2 Infuse; Medtronic). Commonly used particulate onlay techniques include the subperiosteal tunnel technique and direct onlay grafting with or without space maintenance procedures (tenting screws, guided barrier regeneration [GBR]).

SUBPERIOSTEAL TUNNEL GRAFTING

Subperiosteal tunnel grafting is effective for adding small to moderate amounts of bone to augment horizontal alveolar bone defects caused by resorption of the buccal plate. Ideal graft sites include an alveolus that is thinnest at the crest and widens in dimension as it approaches basal bone (ie, buccal plate defect). This particular type of ridge morphology, in addition to being commonplace, is ideal for a tunneled particulate graft as the wider base acts to support the grafted material. Indications for subperiosteal tunnel grafting include sites with sufficient vertical height maintained by the lingual plate and a lingual to buccal sloping alveolar ridge less than 4 mm in crestal width.[41]

Surgical Technique

Local anesthetic containing a vasoconstrictor is used to hydro-dissect the tissue overlying the buccal wall defect (**Fig. 4**A–C). A vertical incision is planned away from the planned graft site in a manner that will allow for access to the graft site and a tension-free closure (see **Fig. 4**E and D). A subperiosteal tunnel is created with the use of a periosteal elevator to elevate the periosteum in the area of the proposed graft. The dissection should not enter the retromolar pad, cross over to the lingual aspect of the alveolus, or violate muscular attachments. Particulate graft is injected into the tunnel with the aid of a 1-mL syringe and digitally molding (see **Fig. 4**F). Demineralized particulate grafts are typically used because of delayed resorption and slower incorporation compared with mineralized particulate grafts. The mesial incision is closed in a tension-free manner with resorbable sutures (see **Fig. 4**G). Patients are advised to avoid mastication of the grafted site and to avoid prosthesis placement over the grafted area for several months because this may displace the graft and accelerate the resorption process (see **Fig. 4**H–K). The graft is typically allowed to consolidate for 3 to 4 months before implant placement. Fibrin sealants have been used to transform the loose particulate into a moldable putty and to minimize particulate migration.[42]

DIRECT PARTICULATE ONLAY GRAFTING

Direct particulate onlay grafting is effective for horizontal deficiencies in the anterior maxilla, in saddle depressions, and in regions with particularly advantageous osseous morphology to contain the particulate graft, such as 3-wall and 4-wall bony defects with an apical bony stop. The use of membranes, although not required, has been shown to decrease particulate graft resorption, especially when used for implant coverage.[43,44] The integrity of direct particulate onlay grafts may be enhanced with the addition of fibrin sealants or protein-based regenerative gels (Emdogain; Straumann, Andover, MA, USA).

Direct Particulate Onlay Grafting Technique

This technique may be used to augment deficient horizontal osseus dimensions before or in conjunction with implant placement (**Fig. 5**A, B). Mucoperiosteal tissue flaps are created, typically with the aid of a releasing incision, to ensure direct visualization of all bony borders of the defect site and to aid in a tension-free closure (see **Fig. 5**C, D; **Fig. 6**D). Particulate graft material is placed within the bony depression and compacted with digital pressure (see **Fig. 5**E, F and **6**H). Demineralized particulate grafts are typically used because of their delayed resorption and slower incorporation times compared with mineralized particulate grafts (see **Fig. 5**G–J). For small to moderate horizontal ridge augmentations, the wound may be closed with or without a resorbable membrane. For moderate to large horizontal ridge augmentations, a slow resorbing or nonresorbable membrane, tenting screws, fibrin sealant, or protein-based regenerative gel may be used to aid in maintaining the graft space. Tension-free closure of the graft site is a key factor to preventing wound dehiscence and graft loss. Additional flap relaxation may be obtained with periosteal releasing incisions and by increasing the length of pre-existing releasing incisions (see **Fig. 6**).

SYMPHYSIS (CHIN) GRAFT

The mandibular symphysis is capable of providing a corticococancellous block graft consisting of primarily D-1 and D-2 bone[24] for horizontal, vertical, and combined grafting to areas requiring alveolar ridge augmentation. The average symphysis is 1-cm thick in its anterior-posterior dimension with a 1.5-mm-thick cortex.[45] The average amount of harvestable bone as reported by Montazem and colleagues[46] was 20.9 (length) × 9.9 (height) × 6.9 mm (depth) with uninterrupted bilateral harvesting. The amount of available bone is

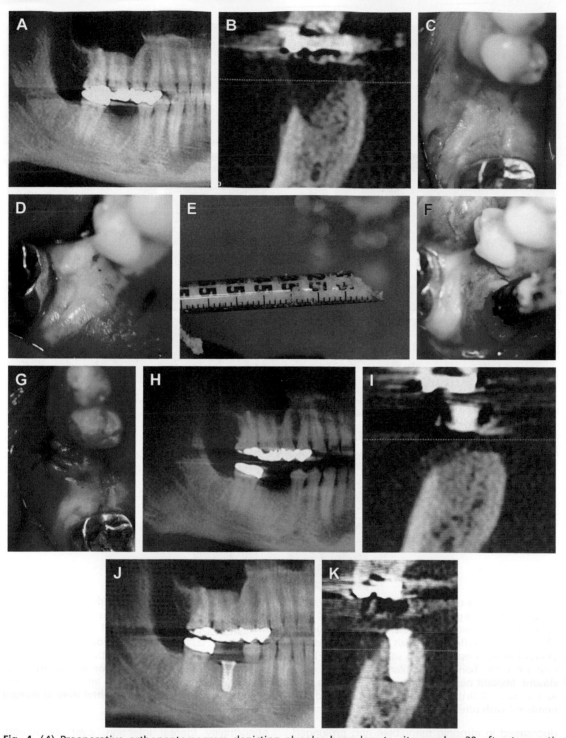

Fig. 4. (*A*) Preoperative orthopantomogram depicting alveolar bone loss to site number 30 after traumatic extraction. (*B*) Coronal image depicting a loss of buccal bone to site number 30. (*C*) Preoperative occlusal view demonstrating loss of the buccal plate to site number 30. (*D*) An incision is made mesial to the graft site, and a periosteal elevator is used to create a subperiosteal tunnel in the region of proposed bone augmentation. (*E*) A 1-mL syringe is modified and used as a carrier for the particulate, demineralized graft. (*F*) Bone is placed within the subperiosteal tunnel using the 1-mL carrier syringe. (*G*) The mesial incision is closed in a tension-free manner with resorbable sutures. (*H*) Graft site after 14 weeks of consolidation. (*I*) Fourteen-week postoperative coronal CBCT image. (*J*) Orthopantomogram obtained 3 months after implant placement site number 30. (*K*) Coronal CBCT image depicting excellent graft retention and implant osseointegration.

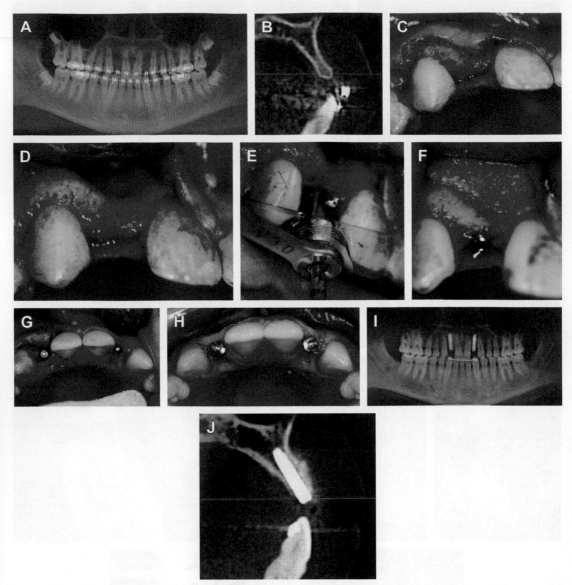

Fig. 5. (*A*) Orthopantomogram depicting a 17-year-old patient near completion of orthodontic therapy with congenitally missing teeth numbers 7 and 10. (*B*) Sagittal view of site number 7 depicting insufficient horizontal bone dimension for implant retention. (*C*) A mucoperiosteal flap is developed with a distal vertical release. (*D*) Mucoperlosteal reflection reveals a saddle depression to site number 7. (*E*) Prefabricated guide in place and initiation of implant osteotomy to site number 7. (*F*) Simultaneous horizontal ridge augmentation with demineralized cadaveric bone and implant placement. (*G*) Periosteal releasing incisions allow for tension-free flap closure. Implant number 10 placed in a flapless fashion due to sufficient bone width. (*H*) Implants uncovered at 4 months. (*I*) Orthopantomogram depicting ideal implant placement. (*J*) Four-month sagittal view of implant number 7 with retention of grafted bone.

decreased in atrophic mandibles and prolonged edentulous regions. Symphysis graft advantages include the ability to obtain a corticocancellous block and increased graft thickness compared with the purely cortical nature and limited thickness of the lateral ramus. Contraindications to symphysis grafting include an anterior mandible with a vertical height of less than 1.5 cm, previous genioplasty, a harvest site with active pathologic abnormality (dental infection, cyst, or tumor), metabolic bone disease, a history of intravenous bisphosphonates, and previous head and neck radiation.

Surgical Technique

Two approaches are used to gain access to the symphysis region, sulcular and vestibular.

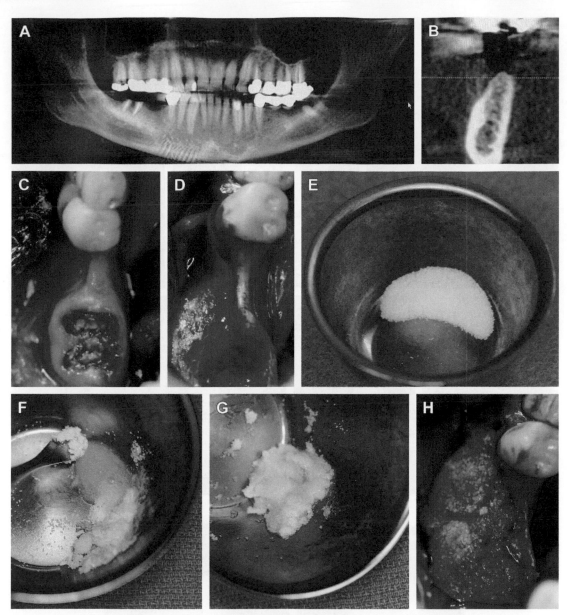

Fig. 6. (*A*) Preoperative orthopantomogram depicting edentulous site number 30 and retained root tips number 31. (*B*) Preoperative coronal view of site number 30 illustrating a significant loss of buccal bone. (*C*) Preoperative occlusal view depicting horizontal ridge atrophy site number 30. (*D*) Root tips site number 31 extracted atraumatically and edentulous site number 30 exposed. (*E*) Particulate bovine bone. (*F*) Addition of Emdogain protein-based regenerative gel. (*G*) Formation of a cohesive moldable graft. (*H*) The Emdogain-bovine graft is placed within the extraction site and edentulous space. (*I*) A collagen membrane is placed over the graft material. (*J*) The site is closed primarily and in a tension-free manner. (*K*) Site 3 weeks postoperatively. (*L*) Site 3 months postoperatively immediately before implant placement. (*M*) Implant are placed in a flapless manner with a CBCT-generated guide. (*N*) Postoperative orthopantomogram. (*O*) Postoperative coronal view implant number 31. (*P*) Postoperative coronal view implant number 30.

Each approach has its potential advantages, disadvantages, as well as relative indications and contraindications. The sulcular approach is associated with an increased risk of gingival recession, and thus, should only be used in patients with a thick soft tissue biotype. Advantages of the sulcular approach include greater access, better visibility, and decreased postoperative paresthesia. Contraindications to the sulcular approach include a thin soft tissue biotype, periodontal disease with

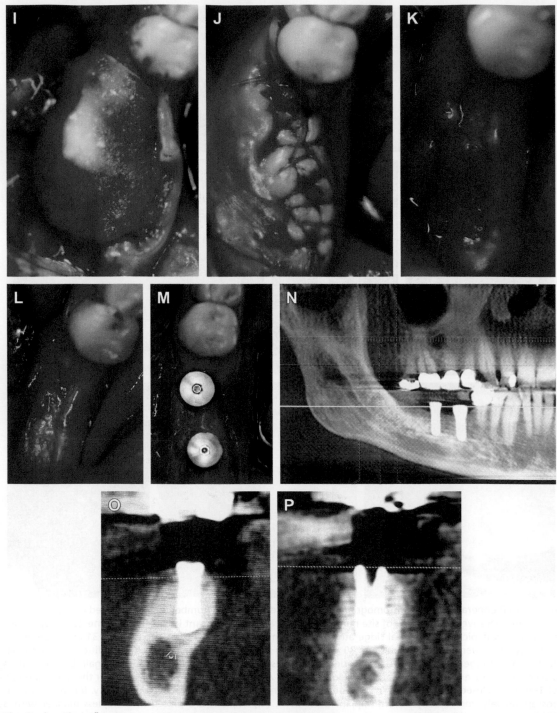

Fig. 6. (*continued*)

evident recession, and gingival or subgingival restorations to the anterior mandibular teeth. The sulcular incision originates along the buccal sulcus of the anterior mandibular teeth and extends to the second premolars/parasymphysis region where bilateral releasing incisions are created, extending from the distobuccal line angles into the vestibule (**Fig. 7**A). A vestibular approach provides more direct access to the symphysis region, but is associated with increased neurosensory disturbances.

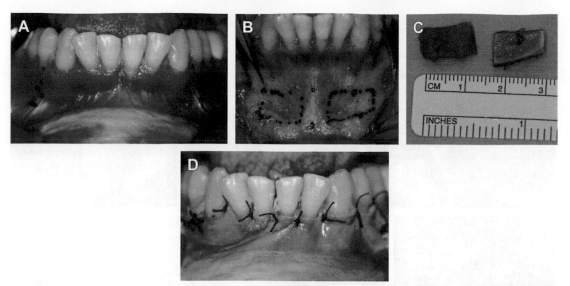

Fig. 7. (*A*) Sulcular approach to the symphysis. Preoperative markings are placed, indicating the location of releasing incisions within the mandibular premolar regions. (*B*) The symphysis is exposed; the mental foramen and nerves are identified, and the sites of graft harvest are marked a minimum of 5 mm from the mental foramen, the apices of the anterior mandibular teeth, and the inferior border of the mandible. A caliber is shown measuring from the anterior aspect of the mental foramen to the posterior aspect of the anticipated graft site. (*C*) Two corticancellous block grafts are harvested. (*D*) Sulcular incision closed with interrupted sutures.

The vestibular incision is initiated 1 cm inferior to the mucogingival junction from first premolar to first premolar and transverses the mentalis muscle.[47]

Once the symphysis is accessed, the mentalis is reflected; the bilateral mental foramen and nerves are visualized and protected, and the inferior border of the anterior mandible is identified. The harvest zone is identified 5 mm lateral to the mental foramen bilaterally, 5 mm superior from the inferior border of the mandible, and 5 mm apical to the anterior teeth roots (see **Fig. 7**B). The average root length of the mandibular central incisor, lateral incisor, canine, and first premolar are 12 mm, 13.5 mm, 15 mm, and 14 mm, respectively.[48,49] In instances where it is difficult to determine the apical extent of the mandibular canine, the superior osteotomy is initiated with an inferior bevel a minimum of 2 cm inferior to the CEJ of the mandibular canine to minimize inadvertent root exposure. Osteotomies may be initiated with any combination of burs, saws, chisels, and/or piezoelectric devices. The graft is harvested atraumatically with the aid of dental elevators and bone chisels with complete preservation of the lingual plate of bone. A monocortical corticancellous graft may be designed unilaterally or bilaterally with or without violating the mandibular midline (see **Fig. 7**C). Careful reapproximation and positioning of the mentalis muscle after graft harvest are key steps to minimizing chin ptosis and postoperative wound dehiscence (see **Fig. 7**D).[50] As it relates to

the development of postoperative chin ptosis, no approach has been shown to be statistically superior to the other.[47]

Complications associated with symphysis grafts include neurosensory disturbances, damage to overlying teeth roots, hematoma formation, wound dehiscence, chin ptosis, and gingival recession (sulcular approach). Temporary paresthesia has been reported between 10% and 76% in the literature, with reports of permanent paresthesia/anesthesia ranging from 13% to 52%.[51–53] Graft resorption rates and total augmentation vary considerably within the literature. Cordaro and colleagues[54] reported resorption of 23.5% for horizontal augmentation and 42% for vertical augmentation. Pikos[24] reported an average gain of 4 to 6 mm of bone (horizontal or vertical) when using symphysis block grafts.

LATERAL RAMUS GRAFT

The lateral ramus/coronoid process graft provides a D-1 cortical graft capable of providing increased overall bone volume with increased length and decreased width compared with a symphysis graft (**Fig. 8**A). Available bone for grafting originates distal to the mesial root of the first molar and extends cephalically to include the coronoid process if necessary. The superior margin of the graft coincides with the external oblique ridge and the inferior margin of the graft extends 10 to 12 mm

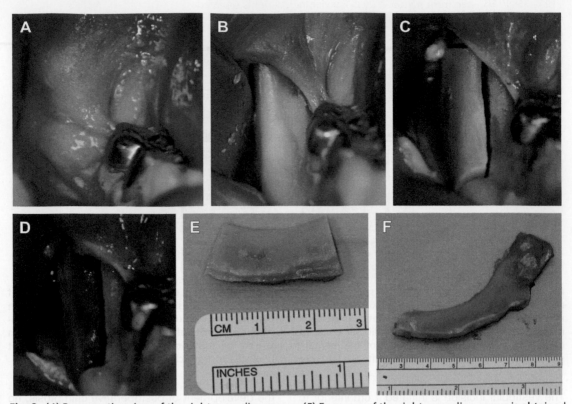

Fig. 8. (*A*) Preoperative view of the right ascending ramus. (*B*) Exposure of the right ascending ramus is obtained via a sulcular incision with continuation of the incision along the external oblique ridge. (*C*) A piezoelectric device is used to create an anterior vertical osteotomy originating at the thickest aspect of the buccal plate (Dal Pont prominence). A posterior vertical osteotomy is placed as far posteriorly as needed. A crestal horizontal osteotomy connects the 2 points while staying lateral to the molar teeth. A round bur or angled saw/piezoelectric attachment may be used to score the inferior aspect of the donor site 4 to 5 mm superior to the mandibular canal to aid in a predictable out-fracture. (*D*) Donor site after ramus harvest. (*E*) A 30 mm × 13 mm × 1.5 mm cortical ramus graft. (*F*) Combined ramus-coronoid graft with the posterior vertical osteotomy extending through the sigmoid notch.

below the external oblique ridge or 4 mm above the mandibular canal. The cortical thickness of an ascending ramus graft varies from 1.0 to 2.5 mm[23] with the thickest area of bone adjacent to the second molar (Dal Pont prominence). The traditional ramus graft originates at the Dal Pont prominence and extends to the third molar region (**Fig. 1**). The traditional ramus graft yields a cortical block measuring 13 mm (vertical) × 30 mm (length) (see **Fig. 8**E).[55] The traditional ramus graft may be extended to the sigmoid notch to include the coronoid process if additional cortical bone is required (see **Fig. 8**F).[23] Overall, the ascending ramus yields more bone than any other intraoral harvest site.

Surgical Technique

A sulcular incision is initiated along the necks of the mandibular molar teeth and is continued posteriorly and laterally along the external oblique ridge. Mucoperiosteal tissue elevation is performed to expose the underlying lateral ramus from the first molar to the ascending ramus (see **Fig. 8**B). Graft markings based on the preoperative workup are made with either electrocautery, a sterile marking pen, or shallow grooves from a bur. Osteotomies are created with any combination of burs (fissured and round), saws (reciprocating and oscillating), and/or piezoelectric devices (see **Fig. 8**C). Piezoelectric devices have the advantage of decreasing inferior alveolar nerve injuries. A crestal osteotomy is initiated medial to the external oblique ridge with care to maintain at least 2 mm of bone lateral to the molar teeth. The anterior vertical osteotomy is initiated just anterior to the thickest prominence of the buccal plate (Dal Pont prominence). The inferior osteotomy is placed 4 mm above the anticipated course of the mandibular canal based on measurements performed during the preoperative workup. The posterior vertical osteotomy is based on the amount of bone required for the recipient site. The posterior osteotomy can extend as far posterior as the sigmoid notch to include the coronoid process, if needed. All osteotomies extend to the marrow space of the mandible, unless the osteotomy extends so far posteriorly that a marrow space cannot be identified. Once all osteotomies are completed, the ascending ramus graft is outfractured and the recipient site is inspected (see **Fig. 8D**). The authors prefer to perform their outfracturing with a large straight elevator instead of a chisel because of the increased tactile sensation and the ability to detect and correct the propagation of aberrant fractures before completing the out-fracture. Inadvertent unroofing of the mandibular canal is treated with careful inspection of the inferior alveolar nerve. Damage to the epineurium is managed by ensuring the nerve is passively positioned within the mandibular canal. Partial or complete severance of the nerve is treated with tension-free reanastomosis with 8-0 Nylon sutures. The donor site is copiously irrigated and closed with resorbable sutures.

Complications associated with lateral ramus grafts include intraoperative bleeding from the inferior alveolar artery or vein, neurosensory disturbance, damage to the molar teeth, hematoma formation, wound dehiscence, infection, unfavorable graft fracture pattern, mandibular fracture, and prolonged trismus. It has been reported that the inferior alveolar nerve is exposed during 10% to 12% of all ramus grafts.[24] Temporary paresthesia has been reported between 0% and 21% in the literature, with reports of permanent paresthesia/anesthesia ranging from 3% to 8.3%.[51,53] Pikos[24] has reported similar graft resorption of ramus grafts compared with symphysis grafts with an average augmentation (horizontal and vertical) of 3 to 4 mm.

TUBEROSITY GRAFT

The maxillary tuberosity is a source of cancellous bone that extends from the distal aspect of the second molar to the posterior aspect of the maxillary alveolus. The average tuberosity yields 1 to 3 mL of uncompressed D-3 or D-4 type bone.[45] The floor of the maxillary sinus forms the superior boundary while the alveolar mucosa forms the inferior boundary. Key anatomic structures associated with tuberosity harvest include the maxillary sinus, the maxillary molars, and the posterior superior alveolar artery (PSA), which is located approximately 15 mm superior to the pterygomaxillary fissure.[56] Maxillary tuberosity volume is diminished in instances with retained third molars, in edentulous sites, and secondary to sinus hyperpneumatization.[57] Indications for tuberosity grafting include socket preservation, reconstruction of three-wall or four-wall dentoalveolar defects, and sinus augmentation. The maxillary tuberosity and associated exostoses may be used as a block onlay graft as an alternative to symphysis or ramus grafting.[9]

Surgical Technique

Exposure of the tuberosity is achieved via an incision directly over the tuberosity, extending from the Hamular notch to the second molar, where a vertical release is used to aid in visualization. Strict adherence to a subperiosteal dissection will minimize exposure and subsequent herniation of the buccal fat pad. Once exposed, tuberosity bone is harvested with the use of rongeurs and curettes while remaining 2 mm from the maxillary sinus and adjacent maxillary molar teeth as measured on preoperative films. After harvest completion, all sharp edges of bone are recontoured and the site is closed with resorbable sutures.

Complications associated with tuberosity grafting include hematoma formation, wound dehiscence, and sinus perforation. Hematoma formation or arterial bleeding from the PSA is rarely encountered and is initially treated with direct compression of the area and close observation until hematoma expansion or bleeding subsides.

Small perforations are treated with primary closure of the mucosa and sinus precautions for 10 days (decongestants, antibiotics, smoking cessation, and avoidance of sneezing). Larger perforations or perforations resulting in fistula formation are treated with buccal fat pad advancement and layered closure techniques often requiring local tissue flap advancements.

RIDGE SPLIT TECHNIQUE

The ridge split or "book bone flap"[58] is used to increase the horizontal alveolar dimensions of an atrophic alveolus. A ridge split involves a crestal incision placed slightly lingually/palatally in the area of the alveolar segment to be augmented. Mucoperiosteal tissue elevation is performed only at the alveolar crest to maintain optimal facial blood supply to the out-fractured segment of the buccal plate. A blind 10- to 12-mm vertical osteotomy is initiated 2 mm from adjacent dental roots while preserving 2 mm of the lingual plate, creating an osteoperiosteal facial flap with at least a 2-mm thickness of facial bone. Care is taken to maintain the 2-mm thickness of lingual/palatal and facial bone as the osteotomy is propagated to preserve the blood supply to the out-fractured segment. The facial bone flap is then out-fractured with a dental elevator or chisel. Dental implants or grafting material is placed within the osseous void. The crestal incision is closed without advancement of the buccal mucosa. If primary closure cannot be obtained, a membrane should be placed to avoid excessive tension of the pedicled facial osteoperiosteal flap. In a report of 500 cases, Jensen and Ellis[58] reported an average horizontal gain of 3 mm when using the ridge split technique. Indications for ridge splitting include edentulous areas with sufficient vertical height for implant placement, edentulous sites with a minimum of 4 mm of horizontal alveolar bone, and regions requiring 2 to 5 mm of horizontal ridge augmentation.[59] Advantages of ridge splitting include predictable horizontal ridge augmentation and the possibility of immediate implant placement. Disadvantages include buccal plate resorption, gingival recession, devitalization of the out-fractured segment with subsequent facial bone loss/resorption, and the lack of ability to gain vertical bone height.[60]

INTERPOSITIONAL BONE GRAFTING

Interpositional bone grafting (IPBG) or "sandwich grafting" is used to increase the vertical alveolar dimensions of a severely atrophic alveolus. IPBG involves exposing the facial/buccal aspect of the bone to be augmented, typically the anterior maxilla or the posterior mandible, and performing bone osteotomies at the site of augmentation.[61] Two vertical osteotomies are placed at the proximal and distal aspect of the atrophic region and a horizontal osteotomy is created a minimum of 3 mm from the inferior alveolar nerve, maxillary sinus, or floor of the nasal cavity to create a mobile transport segment of bone. Care is taken to preserve the attachment of the crestal tissue to the

transport segment and to avoid perforation of the lingual/palatal tissue as this tissue pedicle is a key factor to graft success. The transport segment is raised only as far as the lingual/palatal soft tissue pedicle will allow, typically a maximum of 5 mm within the anterior maxilla[62] and 8 mm within the posterior mandible.[63]

Sources of autogenous or alloplastic cancellous or cortical bone are "sandwiched" between the basal bone and the transport segment and the transport segment is rigidly fixated with bone plates or positional screws (**Fig. 9**).[64] Indications for IPBG include areas requiring only vertical alveolar augmentation, a minimum of 4 mm of bone from the alveolar crest to the mandibular canal, maxillary sinus, and/or nasal cavity and regions with sufficient space for the placement of vertical osteotomies without encroaching on adjacent tooth roots. Advantages of IPBG include a more predictable means of augmentation compared with onlay grafting, minimal resorption provided preservation of the soft tissue pedicle and avoiding overstretching the lingual/palatal tissue, and increased vertical augmentation compared with onlay grafting.[65] Disadvantages of IPBG include a pre-existing minimum alveolar height of 4 to 5 mm, the risk for iatrogenic sinus/nasal cavity perforation and inferior alveolar nerve damage, and the need for a second procedure to remove hardware.

INFERIOR ALVEOLAR NERVE TRANSPOSITION

Inferior alveolar nerve transposition (IANT) is an alternative to grafting within the atrophic posterior mandible to facilitate the placement of dental implants in areas of minimal vertical height. IANT involves exposing the lateral border of the mandible from the mental foramen to the ascending ramus. A round bur is used to unroof the mandibular canal

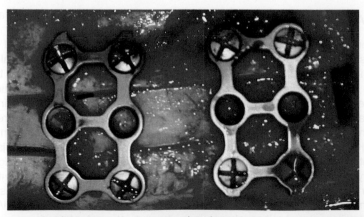

Fig. 9. Interpositional "sandwich" osteotomy depicting the placement of an autogenous cortical graft between the basal bone of the anterior mandible and the transport segment of the mandibular alveolus. Fixation plates are used to maintain the vertical dimension of the graft site.

beginning at the mental foramen. Once the mandibular canal is exposed, the inferior alveolar nerve is lateralized within the soft tissue of the mandibular vestibule and dental implants are placed within the posterior mandible, transversing the empty mandibular canal. Advantages of IANT include the ability to place 8- to 12-mm implants without the need for grafting, no donor site morbidity, and dramatically shortening overall treatment time.[66] Disadvantages of the IANT include the inability to alter the horizontal dimension of the mandible and the high rate of potential complications, such as neurosensory disturbances, mandibular fractures, postoperative pain, and patient's unwillingness to undergo the procedure.[66,67] Reports of neurosensory disturbances vary significantly within the literature. Kan and colleagues[67] reported 52.4% neurosensory disturbances in their patients 41.3 months after IANT.[68]

DISTRACTION OSTEOGENESIS

Distraction osteogenesis (DO) involves the formation of native bone through incremental advancements of a transport segment. Most commercial grade distractors allow for multiplane distraction and, although typically performed for larger edentulous sites, single-tooth unit distractors are available. DO involves the creation of a transport segment with preservation of a lingual and crestal pedicle, similar to IPBG. A vestibular incision is used to expose the surgical site and to allow for preservation of the crestal tissue attachment to the transport segment (**Fig. 10C**). A horizontal osteotomy is initiated to create a transport segment staying a minimum of 2 mm from adjacent teeth roots and 3 mm from the mandibular canal or the maxillary sinus/nasal cavity. Vertical osteotomies are created that are slightly divergent toward the transport segment, thus creating a trapezoidal shape of bone to prevent

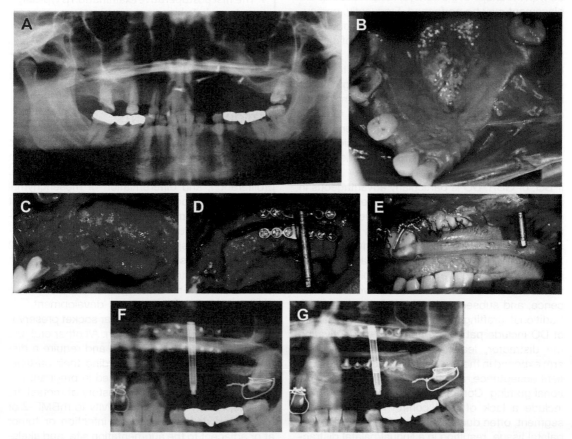

Fig. 10. (*A*) Preoperative orthopantogram demonstrating severe hard tissue loss to the left anterior maxilla. (*B*) Occlusal image depicting significant loss of vertical height to the maxillary alveolus with significant soft tissue loss and scarring. (*C*) Area exposed via a high vestibular incision with care to preserve the crestal and palatal tissue pedicle. (*D*) Alveolar distractor in place with a 2-mm gap created between the transport segment and the underlying basal bone. (*E*) The surgical site is closed and an occlusal splint is placed to control the vector of vertical distraction. (*F*) Immediate postoperative orthopantomogram depicting a 2-mm gap between distractor arms. (*G*) A 4-week orthopantomogram depicting vertical distraction of transport segment.

transport segment interferences during the distraction process. A periosteal elevator is used to mobilize the transport segment. The distraction device is attached to the free-floating transport segment and to the underlying nonosteotomized basal bone. The distractor is activated to test for interferences and then returned to its original starting position, but with a 1- to 2-mm gap (see **Fig. 10**D, F). The site is closed (see **Fig. 10**E) and the distraction process begins after a 5- to 7-day latency period. The latency period allows for the formation of a soft callous within the 1- to 2-mm gap between the transport segment and the nonosteotomized basal bone. The distractor is activated 2 to 4 times per day with a goal of distracting the transport segment 0.5 to 2 mm per day. Once the ideal height of bone is reached, the distractor is left in place for a consolidation period of 4 to 8 weeks (see **Fig. 10**G). At the end of the consolidation period, the distractor is removed. At the time of distractor removal, dependent on the shape of the bone, simultaneous implant placement may be performed. Frequently, particularly with significant distractions, an hourglass shape of bone will be present at the time of distractor removal, with the narrowest portion of bone located at the midpoint between the transport segment and the nonosteotomized segment of basal bone. In these instances, onlay grafting is typically performed at the time of distractor removal, with implant placement 4 to 6 months later.

Indications for DO include the need for significant vertical lengthening of both hard and soft tissue that is traditionally not possible with onlay grafting, IPBG, or GBR. DO is particularly advantageous in areas of previous trauma where there is a significant loss of both bone and soft tissue and where the remaining soft tissue envelope is significantly scarred down (see **Fig. 10**A, B). Advantages of DO include the ability to gain significant hard and soft tissue for extensive defects, the ability to obtain native bone and decreased risk of wound dehiscence, and subsequent infection, compared with traditional grafting procedures.[69] Disadvantages of DO include patient compliance with activating the distractor, leaving the distractor's working arm exposed in the oral cavity for months, poor patient acceptance, and the frequent need for additional grafting. Complications associated with DO include a lack of total control of the transport segment, often due to tethering from the lingual or palatal tissue, resulting in a lingual/palatal distraction vector.[70] Additional complications include infection, relapse, fistula formation at the activation arm, neurosensory disturbances, and the inability to move the transport segment along the entire length of the vertical osteotomies because of the inadvertent creation of convergent walls. **Box 1**

Box 1
Postoperative care following alveolar grafting procedures

- Saline rinses are begun the day after surgery and are continued until complete tissue healing/coverage of the recipient and donor sites occur.

- Oral hygiene is resumed the day after the procedure with the avoidance of the operative sites (recipient and donor) for 2 weeks.

- A soft mechanical diet is recommended for 10 days with avoidance of masticatory forces on the grafted site.

- Oral analgesics and NSAIDs are used for pain control and tissue inflammation, respectively.

- Prosthesis placement is avoided to minimize graft displacement. Alternatively, a soft reline may be performed provided there is no direct pressure on the grafted site.

- The first postoperative examination is typically at 1 week. Subsequent examinations are performed based on the patient's progress and the need for suture and hardware removal.

---

provides postoperative care following all alveolar grafting procedures.

OSTEOINDUCTIVE AGENTS

Recombinant human bone morphogenetic protein-2 (rhBMP-2) is an osteoinductive agent that is known to stimulate angiogenesis, migration, proliferation, and differentiation of mesenchymal stem cells into bone forming cells with resultant de novo bone formation.[71] The effects of rhBMP-2 are locally induced and require a carrier substrate (collagen sponge) for its delivery. rhBMP-2 has been successfully used in combination with other graft materials, including allografts, to provide a space-maintaining osseus substructure and matrix for future bone development.[72,73] rhBMP-2 is approved for alveolar socket preservation and for sinus augmentation. All other oral and maxillofacial uses are off-label and require a discussion with the patient regarding their off-label use. rhBMP-2 should be avoided in pregnant patients, those with active or a history of metastatic disease, allergy or hypersensitivity to rhBMP-2 or associated delivery products, infection or tumor at or adjacent to the augmentation site, and skeletally immature patients. Advantages of rhBMP-2 include de novo bone formation, decreased infection rates, and its osteoinductive properties. Disadvantages of rhBMP-2 include its cost, limited oral and maxillofacial approved applications, and significant edema to the augmentation site.[74]

GUIDED BARRIER REGENERATION

Guided barrier regeneration (GBR) is based on the principle of using membranes to facilitate the formation of bone by maintaining space for bone development while preventing the ingrowth of connective tissue and epithelial cells into the growth site, thus promoting osteogenesis.[75,76] Membranes may be composed of numerous materials and may be either resorbable or nonresorbable. Nonresorbable membranes include titanium mesh, expanded polytetrafluoroethylene (e-PTFE) and TR GTAM (a combination of the 2 with titanium reinforced e-PTFE membrane). Resorbable membranes include collagen, polylactic acid, amniotic membrane, pericardial membrane, and dura mater. The use of GBR is a technically sensitive process that results in predictable horizontal and vertical augmentation of 3 to 6 mm of bone at the time of membrane removal.[75–77] There are 2 main concerns surrounding the use of GBR for alveolar ridge augmentation, the first being of graft resorption after membrane removal and the second being premature membrane exposure. Numerous studies have shown that postaugmentation graft resorption is inhibited only while membranes are in place and that the resorption process begins once the membrane is removed.[78,79] For this reason, many advocate leaving membranes in place for 9[76,77,80] to 12 months[81] with immediate implant placement once the membrane is removed. The second concern when using GBR is of premature membrane exposure (dehiscence). Premature exposure of the membrane frequently leads to contamination of the graft site with oral microorganisms and subsequent infection of the grafted site and inhibition of bone formation.[69,75,81] Premature exposure of membranes is related to surgeon experience, surgical technique, the amount of bone augmented, and the ability to obtain a tension-free closure over the membrane. Most authors agree that a tension-free closure over the membrane is critical to minimize the occurrence of premature membrane exposure (wound dehiscence) and subsequent graft loss. Early membrane exposures frequently lead to complete graft loss, whereas late membrane exposures often lead to only partial graft loss and may be managed with chlorohexadine 0.12% rinses until time for membrane removal.

POSTOPERATIVE CARE

Patients are managed postoperatively with nonsteroidal anti-inflammatory drugs (NSAIDs) and analgesics. Antibiotics are not routinely prescribed. Patients are instructed to masticate on the opposite side of the graft recipient site and to avoid prosthesis placement over the grafted area for several months because this may displace the graft and accelerate the resorption process.

Oral hygiene instructions are reviewed, and the patients are instructed to rinse with salt water daily until complete tissue healing of the recipient and donor sites. The first postoperative examination is typically at 1 week postoperatively and includes a complete neurologic examination involving the distribution of V 3 for cases involving symphysis or ramus harvesting. Additional postoperative visits are based on the invasiveness of the procedure, the patient's progress, and the need for suture and hardware removal.

SUMMARY

Bone augmentation of alveolar defects comprises a wide range of graft materials, donor sites, and surgical approaches. This article summarized essential principles of bone grafting to include basic definitions, bone graft physiology, fixation methods, graft loading and provides a basic foundation for alveolar grafting. An in-depth knowledge of fundamental surgical principles and a comprehensive understanding of available grafting materials, both autogenous and nonautogenous, will enable the oral and maxillofacial surgeon to achieve predictable and sustainable solutions to complex alveolar defects before restoration-driven implant placement.

ACKNOWLEDGMENTS

We would like to thank Bill Winn for providing **Fig. 1** for this article. We would also like to acknowledge Mike Block for his years of tutelage, patience, and for teaching us the art of implant dentistry and grafting.

REFERENCES

1. Parker C. The growth of implant dentistry. The dentist. Surrey (United Kingdom): George Warman Publications; 2012.
2. DiMatteo AM, K. L. Guide to implant dentistry. Inside Dentistry 2014;10:94–100.
3. Medical device excise tax will boost process in the US market for dental implants in 2013. Millenium Research Group; 2013.
4. Rabelo GD, de Paula PM, Rocha FS, et al. Retrospective study of bone grafting procedures before implant placement. Implant Dent 2010;19(4):342–50.
5. Felice P, Iezzi G, Lizio G, et al. Reconstruction of atrophied posterior mandible with inlay technique and mandibular ramus block graft for implant

prosthetic rehabilitation. J Oral Maxillofac Surg 2009;67(2):372–80.

6. Barone A, Covani U. Maxillary alveolar ridge reconstruction with nonvascularized autogenous block bone: clinical results. J Oral Maxillofac Surg 2007; 65(10):2039–46.

7. Mohlhenrich SC, Heussen N, Ayoub N, et al. Three-dimensional evaluation of the different donor sites of the mandible for autologous bone grafts. Clin Oral Investig 2014. [Epub ahead of print].

8. Amrani S, Anastassov GE, Montazem AH. Mandibular ramus/coronoid process grafts in maxillofacial reconstructive surgery. J Oral Maxillofac Surg 2010;68(3):641–6.

9. Tolstunov L. Maxillary tuberosity block bone graft: innovative technique and case report. J Oral Maxillofac Surg 2009;67(8):1723–9.

10. Block MS, Ducote CW, Mercante DE. Horizontal augmentation of thin maxillary ridge with bovine particulate xenograft is stable during 500 days of follow-up: preliminary results of 12 consecutive patients. J Oral Maxillofac Surg 2012;70(6):1321–30.

11. Khan SN, Cammisa FP Jr, Sandhu HS, et al. The biology of bone grafting. J Am Acad Orthop Surg 2005;13:77–86.

12. Kao ST, Scott DD. A review of bone substitutes. Oral Maxillofac Surg Clin North Am 2007;19(4): 513–21, vi.

13. Sittitavornwong S, Gutta R. Bone graft harvesting from regional sites. Oral Maxillofac Surg Clin North Am 2010;22(3):317–30, v–vi.

14. Giannoudis PV, Dinopoulos H, Tsiridis E. Bone substitutes: an update. Injury 2005;36(Suppl 3):S20–7.

15. Piattelli M, Favero GA, Scarano A, et al. Bone reactions to anorganic bovine bone (Bio-Oss) used in sinus augmentation procedures: a histologic long-term report of 20 cases in humans. Int J Oral Maxillofac Implants 1999;14(6):835–40.

16. Carmagnola D, Adriaens P, Berglundh T. Healing of human extraction sockets filled with Bio-Oss. Clin Oral Implants Res 2003;14:137–43.

17. Clozza E, Pea M, Cavalli F, et al. Healing of fresh extraction sockets filled with bioactive glass particles: histological findings in humans. Clin Implant Dent Relat Res 2014;16(1):145–53.

18. Bohner M, Galea L, Doebelin N. Calcium phosphate bone graft substitutes: failures and hopes. J Eur Ceram Soc 2012;32(11):2663–71.

19. Marx RE. Bone and bone graft healing. Oral Maxillofac Surg Clin North Am 2007;19(4):455–66, v.

20. Spagnoli DB, Marx RE. Dental implants and the use of rhBMP-2. Oral Maxillofac Surg Clin North Am 2011;23(2):347–61, vii.

21. Andrade MG, Moreira DC, Dantas DB, et al. Pattern of osteogenesis during onlay bone graft healing. Oral Surg Oral Med Oral Pathol Oral Radiol Endod 2010;110(6):713–9.

22. Ozaki W, Buchman SR. Type of bone related to resorption rate. Plast Reconstr Surg 1998;102(2): 291–9.

23. Verdugo F, Simonian K, Smith McDonald R, et al. Quantitation of mandibular ramus volume as a source of bone grafting. Clin Implant Dent Relat Res 2009;11(Suppl 1):e32–7.

24. Pikos MA. Mandibular block autografts for alveolar ridge augmentation. Atlas Oral Maxillofac Surg Clin North Am 2005;13(2):91–107.

25. Oppenheimer AJ, Tong L, Buchman SR. Craniofacial bone grafting: Wolff's law revisited. Craniomaxillofac Trauma Reconstr 2008;1(1):49–61.

26. Wood RA, Mealey BL. Histologic comparison of healing after tooth extraction with ridge preservation using mineralized versus demineralized freeze-dried bone allograft. J Periodontol 2012;83(3):329–36.

27. Block MS, Jackson WC. Techniques for grafting the extraction site in preparation for dental implant placement. Atlas Oral Maxillofac Surg Clin North Am 2006;14(1):1–25.

28. Scardina GA, Carini F, Noto F, et al. Microcirculation in the healing of surgical wounds in the oral cavity. Int J Oral Maxillofac Surg 2013;42(1):31–5.

29. LaTrenta GS, McCarthy JG, Breitbart AS, et al. The role of rigid skeletal fixation in bone-graft augmentation of the craniofacial skeleton. Plast Reconstr Surg 1989;84(4):578–88.

30. Breine U, Branemark PI. Reconstruction of alveolar jaw bone. An experimental and clinical study of immediate and preformed autologous bone grafts in combination with osseointegrated implants. Scand J Plast Reconstr Surg 1980;14(1):23–48.

31. Bell RB, Blakey GH, White RP, et al. Staged reconstruction of the severely atrophic mandible with autogenous bone graft and endosteal implants. J Oral Maxillofac Surg 2002;60(10):1135–41.

32. Rubin CT, Lanyon LE. Regulation of bone formation by applied dynamic loads. J Bone Joint Surg Am 1984;66(3):397–402.

33. Araujo MG, da Silva JC, de Mendonca AF, et al. Ridge alterations following grafting of fresh extraction sockets in man. A randomized clinical trial. Clin Oral Implants Res 2014. [Epub ahead of print].

34. Tan WL, Wong TL, Wong MC, et al. A systematic review of post-extractional alveolar hard and soft tissue dimensional changes in humans. Clin Oral Implants Res 2012;23(Suppl 5):1–21.

35. Vittorini Orgeas G, Clementini M, De Risi V, et al. Surgical techniques for alveolar socket preservation: a systematic review. Int J Oral Maxillofac Implants 2013;28(4):1049–61.

36. Van der Weijden F, Dell'Acqua F, Slot DE. Alveolar bone dimensional changes of post-extraction sockets in humans: a systematic review. J Clin Periodontol 2009;36(12):1048–58.

37. Ten Heggeler JM, Slot DE, Van der Weijden GA. Effect of socket preservation therapies following tooth extraction in non-molar regions in humans: a systematic review. Clin Oral Implants Res 2011; 22(8):779–88.

38. Horowitz R, Holtzclaw D, Rosen PS. A review on alveolar ridge preservation following tooth extraction. J Evid Based Dent Pract 2012;12(3):149–60.

39. Barone A, Ricci M, Tonelli P, et al. Tissue changes of extraction sockets in humans: a comparison of spontaneous healing vs. ridge preservation with secondary soft tissue healing. Clin Oral Implants Res 2013;24:1231–7.

40. Iasella JM, Greenwell H, Miller RL, et al. Ridge preservation with freeze-dried bone allograft and a collagen membrane compared to extraction alone for implant site development—a clinical and histologic study in humans. J Periodontol 2003;74: 990–9.

41. Block MS. Horizontal ridge augmentation using particulate bone. Atlas Oral Maxillofac Surg Clin North Am 2006;14(1):27–38.

42. Mordenfeld A, Johansson CB, Albrektsson T, et al. A randomized and controlled clinical trial of two different compositions of deproteinized bovine bone and autogenous bone used for lateral ridge augmentation. Clin Oral Implants Res 2014;25(3): 310–20.

43. Park SH, Lee KW, Oh TJ, et al. Effect of absorbable membranes on sandwich bone augmentation. Clin Oral Implants Res 2008;19(1):32–41.

44. Fu JH, Oh TJ, Benavides E, et al. A randomized clinical trial evaluating the efficacy of the sandwich bone augmentation technique in increasing buccal bone thickness during implant placement surgery: I. Clinical and radiographic parameters. Clin Oral Implants Res 2014;25(4):458–67.

45. Marx RE, Stevens MR. Atlas of oral and extraoral bone harvesting. Hanover Park (IL): Quintessence Pub; 2010.

46. Montazem A, Valauri DV, St-Hilaire H, et al. The mandibular symphysis as a donor site in maxillofacial bone grafting: a quantitative anatomic study. J Oral Maxillofac Surg 2000;58(12):1368–71.

47. Gapski R, Wang H, Misch CE. Management of incision design in symphysis graft procedures—a review of the literature. J Oral Implantol 2001;27: 134–42.

48. Sicher H, DuBrul EL. Oral anatomy. 6th edition. St Louis (MO): C. V. Mosby; 1975.

49. Berkovitz BK, Holland GR, Moxham BJ. Oral anatomy histology and embryology. 3rd edition. China: Mosby; 2005.

50. Noia CF, Rodriguez-Chessa JG, Ortega-Lopes R, et al. Prospective study of soft tissue contour changes following chin bone graft harvesting. Int J Oral Maxillofac Surg 2012;41(2):176–9.

51. Clavero J, Lundgren S. Ramus or chin grafts for maxillary sinus inlay and local onlay augmentation-comparison of donor site morbidity and complication. Clin Implant Dent Relat Res 2003;5(3):154–60.

52. Chiapasco M, Abati S, Romeo E, et al. Clinical outcome of autogenous bone blocks or guided bone regeneration with e-PTFE membranes for the reconstruction of narrow edentulous ridges. Clin Oral Implants Res 1999;10(4):278–88.

53. Silva FM, Cortez AL, Moreira RW, et al. Complications of intraoral donor site for bone grafting prior to implant placement. Implant Dent 2006;15(4):420–6.

54. Cordaro L, Amade DS, Cordaro M. Clinical results of alveolar ridge augmentation with mandibular block bone grafts in partially edentulous patients prior to implant placement. Clin Oral Implants Res 2002; 13:103–11.

55. Li KK, Schwartz HC. Mandibular body bone in facial plastic and reconstructive surgery. Laryngoscope 1996;106(4):504–6.

56. Choi J, Park HS. The clinical anatomy of the maxillary artery in the pterygopalatine fossa. J Oral Maxillofac Surg 2003;61(1):72–8.

57. Gapski R, Satheesh K, Cobb CM. Histomorphometric analysis of bone density in the maxillary tuberosity of cadavers: a pilot study. J Periodontol 2006; 77(6):1085–90.

58. Jensen OT, Ellis E. The book flap: a technical note. J Oral Maxillofac Surg 2008;66(5):1010–4.

59. Jensen OT. The osteoperiosteal flap: a simplified approach to alveolar bone reconstruction. Hanover Park (IL): Quintessence; 2010.

60. Jensen OT, Cullum DR, Baer D. Marginal bone stability using 3 different flap approaches for alveolar split expansion for dental implants: a 1-year clinical study. J Oral Maxillofac Surg 2009;67(9):1921–30.

61. Pelo S, Boniello R, Gasparini G, et al. Horizontal and vertical ridge augmentation for implant placement in the aesthetic zone. Int J Oral Maxillofac Surg 2007; 36(10):944–8.

62. Jensen OT, Kuhlke L, Bedard JF, et al. Alveolar segmental sandwich osteotomy for anterior maxillary vertical augmentation prior to implant placement. J Oral Maxillofac Surg 2006;64(2):290–6.

63. Jensen OT. Alveolar segmental "sandwich" osteotomies for posterior edentulous mandibular sites for dental implants. J Oral Maxillofac Surg 2006;64(3): 471–5.

64. Kawakami PY, Dottore AM, Bechara K, et al. Alveolar osteotomy associated with resorbable non-ceramic hydroxylapatite or intra-oral autogenous bone for height augmentation in posterior mandibular sites: a split-mouth prospective study. Clin Oral Implants Res 2013;24(9):1060–4.

65. Block MS, Haggerty CJ. Interpositional osteotomy for posterior mandible ridge augmentation. J Oral Maxillofac Surg 2009;67(11 Suppl):31–9.

66. Bovi M. Mobilization of the inferior alveolar nerve with simultaneous implant insertion: a new technique. Case report. Int J Periodontics Restorative Dent 2005;25(4):375–83.

67. Kan JY, Lozada JL, Goodacre CJ, et al. Endosseous implant placement in conjunction with inferior alveolar nerve transposition: an evaluation of neurosensory disturbance. Int J Oral Maxillofac Implants 1997;12(4):463–71.

68. Proussaefs P. Vertical alveolar ridge augmentation prior to inferior alveolar nerve repositioning: a patient report. Int J Oral Maxillofac Implants 2005; 20(2):296–301.

69. Chiapasco M, Romeo E, Casentini P, et al. Alveolar distraction osteogenesis vs. vertical guided bone regeneration for the correction of vertically deficient edentulous ridges: a 1–3-year prospective study on humans. Clin Oral Implants Res 2004;15:82–95.

70. Robiony M, Toro C, Stucki-McCormick SU, et al. The "FAD" (Floating Alveolar Device): a bidirectional distraction system for distraction osteogenesis of the alveolar process. J Oral Maxillofac Surg 2004; 62(9 Suppl 2):136–42.

71. Wikesjo UM, Huang YH, Polimeni G, et al. Bone morphogenetic proteins: a realistic alternative to bone grafting for alveolar reconstruction. Oral Maxillofac Surg Clin North Am 2007;19(4):535–51, vi–vii.

72. Jovanovic SA, Hunt DR, Bernard GW, et al. Long-term functional loading of dental implants in rhBMP-2 induced bone. A histologic study in the canine ridge augmentation model. Clin Oral Implants Res 2003;14:793–803.

73. Fiorellini JP, Howell TH, Cochran D, et al. Randomized study evaluating recombinant human bone morphogenetic protein-2 for extraction socket augmentation. J Periodontol 2005;76:605–13.

74. Davies SD, Ochs MW. Bone morphogenetic proteins in craniomaxillofacial surgery. Oral Maxillofac Surg Clin North Am 2010;22(1):17–31.

75. Simion M, Baldoni M, Rossi P, et al. A comparative study of the effectiveness of e-PTFE membranes with and without early exposure during the healing period. Int J Periodontics Restorative Dent 1994; 14(2):166–80.

76. Simion M, Trisi P, Piattelli A. Vertical ridge augmentation using a membrane technique associated with osseointegrated implants. Int J Periodontics Restorative Dent 1994;14(6):496–511.

77. Artzi Z, Dayan D, Alpern Y, et al. Vertical ridge augmentation using xenogenic material supported by a configured titanium mesh: clinicohistopathologic and histochemical study. Int J Oral Maxillofac Implants 2003;18(3):440–6.

78. Rasmusson L, Meredith N, Kahnberg KE, et al. Effects of barrier membranes on bone resorption and implant stability in onlay bone grafts. An experimental study. Clin Oral Implants Res 1999;10(4): 267–77.

79. Jensen OT, Greer RO Jr, Johnson L, et al. Vertical guided bone-graft augmentation in a new canine mandibular model. Int J Oral Maxillofac Implants 1995;10(3):335–44.

80. Buser D, Dhalin C, Schenk R. Guided bone regeneration in implant dentistry. Chicago: Quintessence; 1994.

81. Tinti C, Parma-Benfenati S. Vertical ridge augmentation: surgical protocol and retrospective evaluation of 48 consecutively inserted implants. Int J Periodontics Restorative Dent 1998;18(5):434–43.

Complex Bone Augmentation in Alveolar Ridge Defects

Alan S. Herford, DDS, MD[a], Katina Nguyen, DDS[b],*

KEYWORDS

- Alveolar bone • Bone augmentation • Bone graft • Implants • Onlay block graft
- Distraction osteogenesis • Guided bone regeneration • Osteoperiosteal flap split ridge procedure

KEY POINTS

- The current gold standard for bone grafting is autogenous bone, due to its biocompatibility, lack of antigenicity, osteoconductive, and osteoinducive properties.
- Radiography using cone-beam computed tomography for complex defects is useful in determining the amount of bone available and what bone augmentation technique will be needed.
- Many options for treatment of alveolar ridge defects are available, including varying surgical techniques as well as bone graft options.

INTRODUCTION

With the advancement of reconstructive techniques, implants have become an increasingly available option for replacing missing dentition in patients. One of the challenges with implant placement is an unfavorable local condition of the alveolar ridge due to atrophy, which may cause insufficient bone volume in the horizontal and/or vertical dimensions. Many options for treatment of alveolar ridge defects are available, including varying surgical techniques as well as bone graft options. The technique and type of material used depend on the geometry and location of the defect.

On the loss of dentition, there is significant change in the alveolar bone due to the activity of osteoclasts during bone remodeling. The most significant change occurs during the 3 months after loss of dentition and can continue over time with an additional loss of 11% of volumetric bone.[1] A study by Ashman showed that there is an average loss of 40% to 60% of the total bone height and width within the first 2 to 3 years.[2] The greatest bone resorption occurs in the horizontal plane, which leads to a considerable loss of alveolar width.[1]

Various factors can lead to a complex or challenging defect. These characteristics include the location of the defect as well as the size and shape of the defect. Close proximity of anatomic structures such as the inferior alveolar nerve or maxillary sinus may increase the complexity of the reconstruction. Patient factors such as poor healing states or unsuccessful previous surgeries can transform a relatively straightforward defect to a more challenging one.

EVIDENCE

Multiple extensive reviews of the literature have been performed in an attempt to provide a more evidence-based approach for grafting of defects.[2–6] One such review by Aghaloo and Moy[7] looked at which hard tissue augmentation techniques are the most successful in furnishing bony

[a] Department of Oral and Maxillofacial Surgery, Loma Linda University, 11092 Anderson Street, Loma Linda, CA 92350, USA; [b] Department of Oral and Maxillofacial Surgery, Loma Linda University, 11092 Anderson Street, Loma Linda, CA 92350, USA
* Corresponding author.
E-mail address: knguyen@llu.edu

Oral Maxillofacial Surg Clin N Am 27 (2015) 227–244
http://dx.doi.org/10.1016/j.coms.2015.01.003
1042-3699/15/$ – see front matter © 2015 Elsevier Inc. All rights reserved.

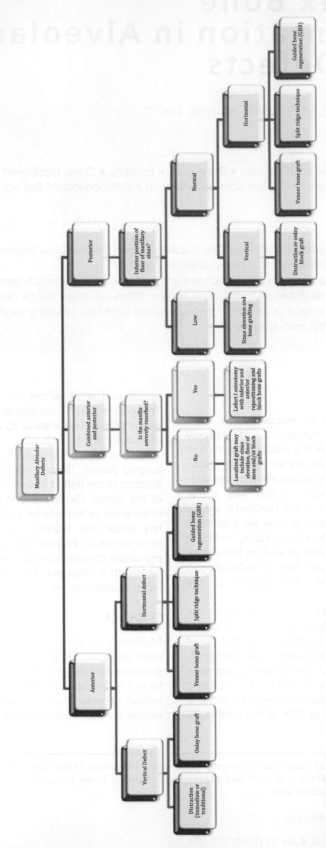

Fig. 1. Maxillary bone augmentation algorithm.

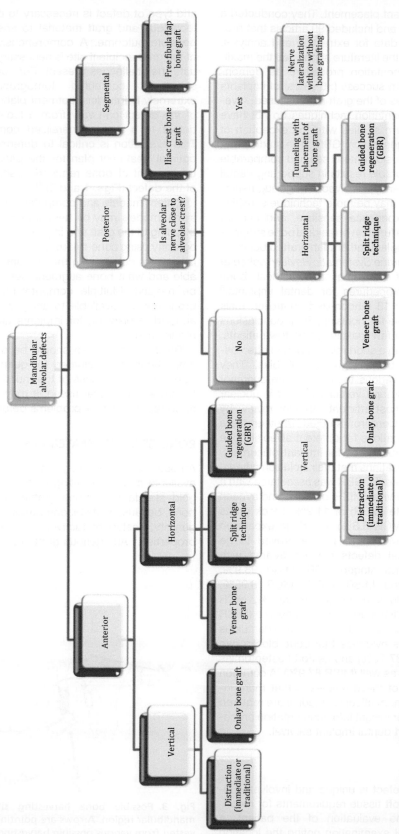

Fig. 2. Mandibular bone augmentation algorithm.

support for implant placement. They conducted a systemic review and included 90 articles that provided sufficient data for extraction and analysis. They found that the literature supported the maxillary sinus augmentation procedure as demonstrating long-term success (>5 years) of implants placed regardless of the graft material used. Alveolar ridge augmentation techniques do not have detailed long-term studies with the exception of guided bone regeneration (GBR). The studies that did meet the inclusion criteria seemed comparable and yielded favorable results in supporting dental implants. Importantly, the alveolar ridge augmentation procedures may be more technique sensitive and operator-experience sensitive, and implant survival may be a function of residual bone supporting the dental implant rather than grafted bone.

A recent Cochrane Systematic Review looked at the efficacy of horizontal and vertical bone augmentation procedures for dental implants.[8] They found only 13 randomized controlled trials that were suitable for inclusion. Their conclusions were based on a few trials including few patients, sometimes having a short follow-up, and often being judged to be a high risk of bias. They concluded that various techniques can augment bone horizontally and vertically, but it is unclear which are the most efficient. Another review by Milinkovic and Cordaro[9] studied whether there are specific indications for different alveolar bone augmentation procedures for implant placement. Sixty-eight publications met their inclusion criteria. For horizontal defects, GBR was associated with a mean implant survival (MISR) of 100% and a mean complication rate (MCR) of 11.9%. Block grafts (MISR 98.4%, MCR 6.3%) and ridge expansion (MISR 97.4%, MCR 6.8%) have proved to be effective. Vertical defects can be treated with simultaneous and staged GBR (MISR 98.9%, MCR 13.1% and MISR 100%, MCR 6.95%, respectively), block grafts (MISR 96.3%, MCR 8.1%), and distraction osteogenesis (MISR 98.2%, MCR 22.4%). In completely edentulous patients, there is evidence that bone blocks can be used (MISR 87.75%) and Le Fort I osteotomies can be effective as well (MISR 87.9%). A common theme from all of these studies is that more in-depth, long-term, multicenter studies are required to provide further insight into augmentation procedures to support dental implant survival.

EVALUATION

Each alveolar defect is unique and involves specific hard and soft tissue requirements for reconstruction. In the evaluation of the patient, a stepwise clinical examination noting the location and type of defect is necessary to determine the technique and graft material to ensure the best possible outcome. A comprehensive evaluation of the graft recipient site is necessary to fully evaluate the challenges present. For complex reconstructions, computed tomography (CT) is extremely helpful for treatment planning. The size of the defect can vary from a localized minimal defect to a more generalized complex defect. This evaluation is critical to determine the most optimal treatment plan for the patient, including the amount of bone required based on the size of the defect (**Figs. 1** and **2**).[10]

Patient models and computer-guided 3-dimensional models may be helpful in the preoperative planning of the graft and implant placement. Radiography using cone-beam CT for complex defects is useful in determining the amount of bone available and what bone augmentation technique will be needed. Multiple computer-based software programs are available to analyze the CT scans and aid in planning for implants and bone graft requirements.

The soft tissue also should be assessed. The area should be evaluated for quantity of keratinized tissue, thickness of the mucosa, as well as the presence of scar tissue. It may be preferable to correct soft tissue problems before grafting.

BONE GRAFTING MATERIALS

Autogenous grafts, allografts, and xenografts are available as bone grafting materials. The current gold standard for bone grafting is autogenous bone, because of its biocompatibility, lack of antigenicity, osteoconductive, and osteoinducive properties.[2] Autogenous grafts can be harvested

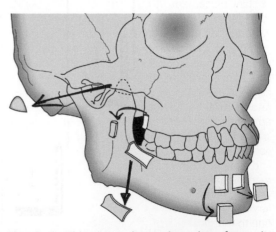

Fig. 3. Possible bone harvesting sites from the mandibular region. Arrows are pointing to bone harvested from various possible harvesting sites.

from various locations. Bone obtained from these sites varies in volume composition, contour characteristics, and embryologic origin. Autogenous grafts are the most predictable graft materials used for reconstruction of complex alveolar defects. Autogenous bone is often the bone graft chosen for complex defects, because of its biocompatibility, lack of antigenicity, osteoconductive, and osteoinducive properties.[11] Alveolar defects can be restored by corticocancellous

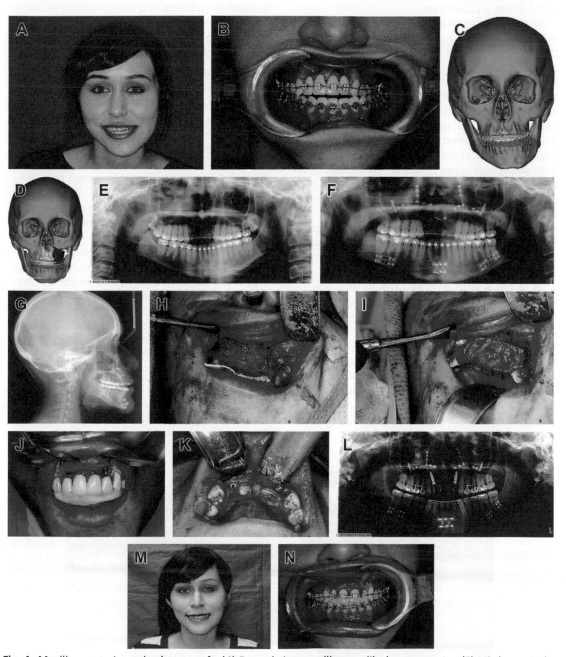

Fig. 4. Maxillary anterior onlay bone graft. (*A*) Frontal view maxilla mandibular asymmetry. (*B*) Missing anterior teeth with bone defect, occlusal view. (*C*) Medical modeling preoperative frontal view: note the anterior maxillary defect. (*D*) Medical modeling final planned frontal view. (*E*) Preoperative panoramic radiograph. (*F*) Panoramic radiograph after orthognathic surgery. (*G*) Lateral radiograph before anterior maxillary grafting. (*H*) Iliac crest onlay bone graft in place covered with particulate bone graft. (*I*) Collagen membrane covering graft. (*J*) Implants in place. (*K*) Grafted bone and implants. (*L*) Postoperative panoramic radiograph with implants in place. (*M*) Postoperative frontal view. (*N*) Postoperative occlusion.

blocks, particular marrow cancellous marrow bone, and cortical grafts harvested from the mandible, maxilla, and cranium. Various bone grafts provides proteins, bone-enhancing substrates, minerals, and vital bone cells to the recipient site, which would enhance the overall success of the grafting procedure.

Autogenous bone can be harvested from intraoral or extraoral sites with their risks of morbidity related to the harvest site.[12] Careful consideration of the harvest site must be factored in, such as location of the recipient bed, the quality and quantity of the required bone graft, and the potential for surgical complications.[3] Advantages of local grafts include the proximity of the donor and recipient sites, convenient surgical access, avoidance of a surgical scar, and decreased operative and anesthesia time.[13] Local grafts are most commonly harvested from the mandible and offer some advantages over distant donor sites, including convenience of surgical access and proximity of the donor and recipient sites (**Fig. 3**). Intraoral donor grafts are typically associated with less resorption than iliac crest, proximal tibia, and rib grafts. The main disadvantage of intraoral sites is the limited amount of bone that can be harvested for reconstruction. When larger quantities of one are required, the iliac crest and proximal tibia are the preferred sites for bone harvest. The iliac crest is most often used for major jaw reconstruction because of its properties and the amount of bone available. It does have disadvantages, including the need for hospitalization, general anesthesia, and alteration of ambulation.

Bone morphogenic protein (rhBMP-2) is approved for localized alveolar defects. Studies have been performed that have shown that the use of bone morphogenic protein (BMP) is useful in the enhancement of bone formation when used in conjunction with bone grafting procedures.[14] This protein is combined with an absorbable collagen sponge and induces bone formation through recruitment and differentiation of mesenchymal stem cells.

SURGICAL PROCEDURES

Surgical procedures, including onlay block grafts, interpositional grafts, GBR, and various combinations of techniques, are available. Free tissue microvascular grafts may be considered for extensive defects involving missing hard and soft tissue as well as patients undergoing radiation therapy.

Before placing grafts to reconstruct the defect, the recipient site should be prepared by carefully removing granulation tissue and eliminating any sharp bony margins. It is encouraged to perforate the underlying cortex before placing the graft to improve integration of the graft.

Implants may be placed simultaneous with the grafting or secondarily. Most studies suggest that the delayed placement of implants should be considered to be more predictable than immediate placement.[15] If implants are placed at the time of grafting, the basal, ungrafted bone should provide stability of the implants without relying on the grafted bone to provide stability.

Onlay Block Grafting

Bone can be harvested from various sites and used to reconstruct alveolar defects (**Figs. 4–8**). Depending on how block grafts are shaped and

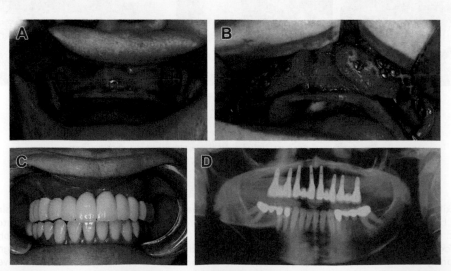

Fig. 5. Localized maxillary combined graft with sinus lift. (*A*) Maxillary defect with previous sinus surgery. (*B*) Onlay graft secured in place. (*C*) Implant restoration, 5 years postoperatively. (*D*) Five-year postoperative radiograph.

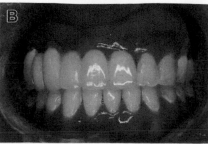
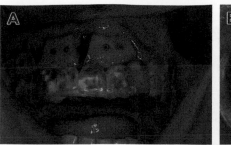

Fig. 6. Maxillary anterior veneer graft. (*A*) Onlay graft secured in place. (*B*) Implant restored with restoration 10 years later.

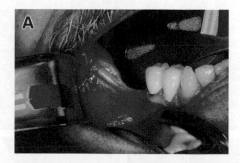

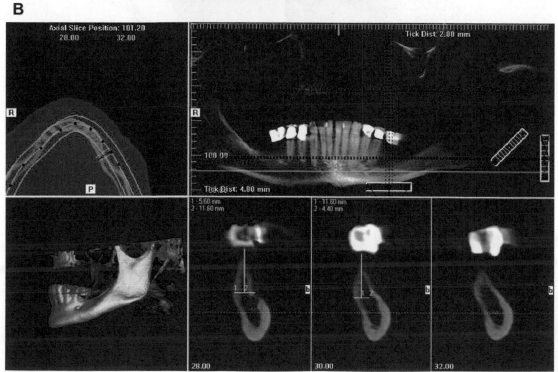

Fig. 7. Mandibular veneer graft. (*A*) Preoperative defect. (*B*) Preoperative CT scans. (*C*) Preoperative CT scans. (*D*) Ramus graft secured in place. (*E*) Graft covered with bovine bone. (*F*) Collagen membrane covering graft. (*G*) Tension-free closure. (*H*) Ramus graft on contralateral side. (*I*) Implant in place. (*J*) Implant in grafted bone. (*K*) Postoperative panoramic radiograph.

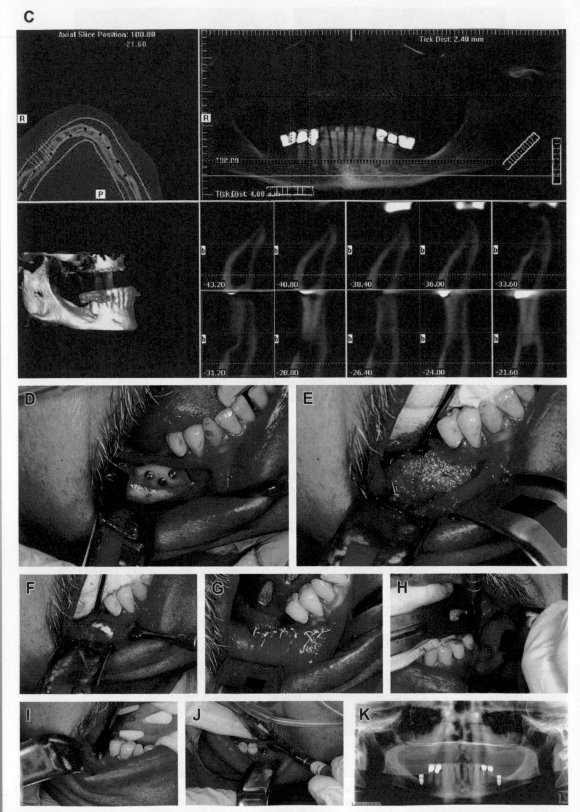

Fig. 7. (continued)

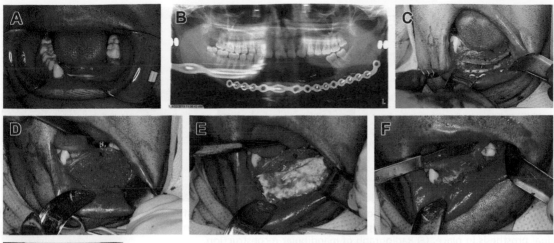

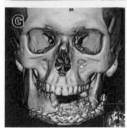

Fig. 8. Mandibular anterior onlay bone graft. (*A*) Patient with fibula free flap reconstruction with inadequate bone height. (*B*) Preoperative radiograph. (*C*) Placement of corticocancellous graft superiorly. (*D*) Placement of cancellous bone between the bone superior and inferiorly. (*E*) Placement of collagen membrane over graft. (*F*) Tension-free closure over graft. (*G*) Postoperative bone graft.

used to restore the defect, they may be in the form of inlays, veneers, onlays, or saddle grafts. Ridge defects that have adequate vertical height but are too narrow may be restored with a veneer graft. Deficient alveolar ridges that require both horizontal and vertical augmentation may be restored with a saddle graft. The grafts must have a cortical portion that will allow screws to be placed to prevent the graft from moving during healing. These grafts are revascularized and replaced with host bone. There is a process of resorption and replacement of bone. Block grafts take longer to integrate than cancellous gone grafts, and a staged surgical approach is more predictable than placing implants in conjunction with the graft. Placing the implant simultaneously with the graft may be considered if there is sufficient basal bone to provide primary stability of the implant without relying on support from the grafted bone.[16]

Distraction Osteogenesis

Distraction osteogenesis can be used to regenerate missing hard and soft tissue (**Fig. 9**).[17,18] Distraction osteogenesis relies on the body's ability to generate bone as 2 segments of bone are "distracted" apart. The osteotomies are created, and the distraction device is placed. Typically there is a latency phase of 1 week where a fibrovascular bridge is formed in the osteotomy site. This fibrovascular bridge provides a template to generate new bone as the segments are distracted apart during the activation phase. Once the desired distraction has occurred, the device is left in place for a period of time. Once consolidation has occurred, the distraction device can be removed and implants can be placed.

Immediate distraction or the "sandwich technique" is similar to distraction osteogenesis, but the application of the distractor is not necessary (**Figs. 10** and **11**).[19] The osteotomy is the same as the traditional alveolar distraction. The transported segment is placed into the desired location and stabilized, creating a well-defined pocket to place a bone graft and leading to predictable healing. By maintaining the soft tissue attached to the transported segment of bone, the blood supply remains, which is different than placing an onlay block graft and requiring revascularization of the graft along the crest of the alveolus; this may lead to less resorption in this area.[20]

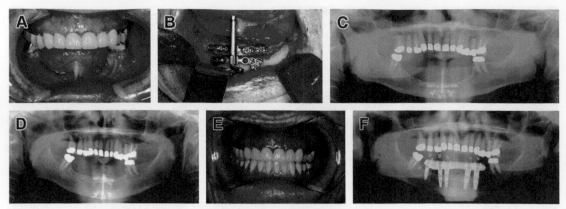

Fig. 9. Mandibular anterior distraction. (*A*) Mandibular anterior defect after tumor removal. (*B*) Placement of alveolar distraction device. (*C*) Postoperative radiograph before activation. (*D*) Radiograph after activation. (*E*) Final prosthesis in place. (*F*) Radiograph of mandibular reconstruction.

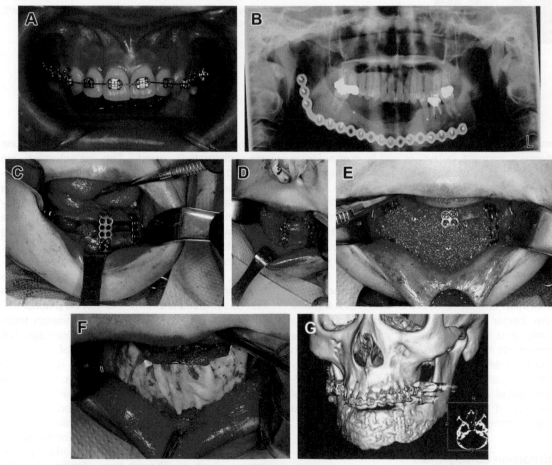

Fig. 10. Mandibular anterior distraction. (*A*) Mandibular defect after tumor removal. (*B*) Radiograph of significant mandibular defect. (*C*) Sandwich osteotomy created and secured superiorly approximately 1 cm. (*D*) Placement of bone graft and growth factor between the bone segments. (*E*) Placement of graft over the top of the osteotomy. (*F*) Collagen membrane covering graft. (*G*) Postoperative mandibular reconstruction.

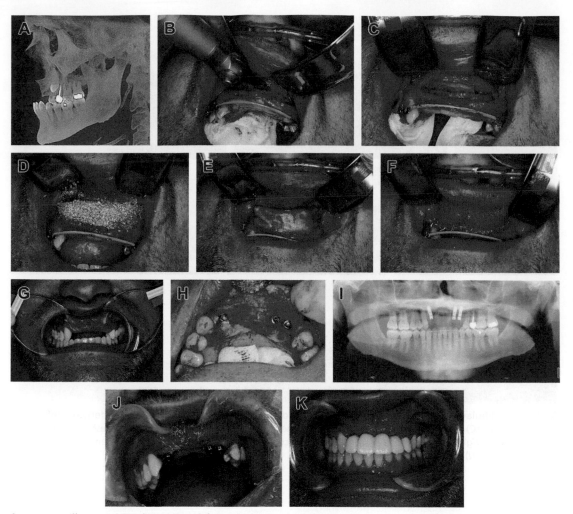

Fig. 11. Maxillary anterior distraction. (*A*) Preoperative radiograph with anterior maxillary defect. (*B*) Creation of osteotomy. (*C*) Immediate distraction of transported segment and placement of ramus bone graft interposition-ally. (*D*) Coverage with bovine xenografts. (*E*) Coverage of graft with collagen membrane. (*F*) Tension-free closure. (*G*) Grafted maxilla before implants. (*H*) Placement of 3 implants. (*I*) Radiograph after implant placement. (*J*) Healing abutments on implants placed. (*K*) Interim prosthesis in place.

Guided Bone Regeneration

GBR techniques use a particulate graft with an overlying membrane that promotes stabilization of the graft material and protects the healing graft from competing, nonosteogenic cells (**Figs. 12** and **13**). This membrane may be resorbable or nonresorbable. For horizontal bone augmenta-tions, the use of membranes combined with par-ticulate autogenous bone has led to increased thickness of the alveolar ridge.[21,22] Vertical aug-mentations are much more technique-sensitive and less predictable.[23] For larger, more complex alveolar defects, onlay grafting is more predict-able.[24] GBR with titanium mesh can also be used for localized ridge augmentation.[25]

Osteoperiosteal Flap Split Ridge Procedure

The osteoperiosteal flap ridge split technique is performed for horizontal augmentation of narrow ridges that otherwise would not be suitable for implant placement. This technique consists of splitting the vestibular and buccal cortical plate and further opening the space with osteo-tomes.[26–28] This technique has had a success rate of 98% to 100% according to previous studies that have performed it.[1]

Maxillary Sinus Elevation and Grafting

The maxillary sinus can be predictably elevated and grafted with a variety of materials (**Fig. 14**).

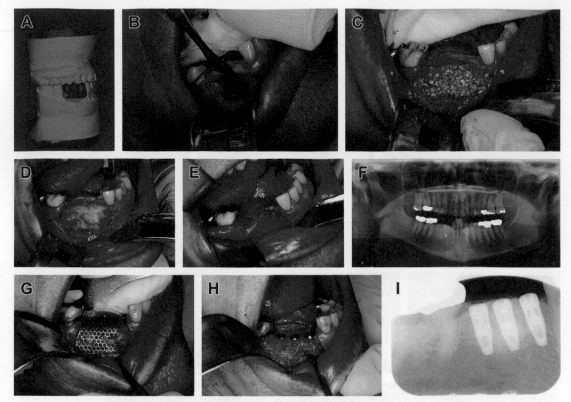

Fig. 12. Mandibular posterior GBR. (*A*) Preoperative models with ideal tooth location. (*B*) Underlying defect after tumor removal. (*C*) Placement of graft over titanium mesh. (*D*) Collagen membrane over mesh. (*E*) Tension-free closure. (*F*) Radiograph after mesh placement. (*G*) Uncovering of titanium mesh. (*H*) Placement of osteointegrated implants. (*I*) Radiograph of implants in place.

This technique is helpful for patients who have a pneumatized sinus and inadequate bone to place implants. Placing a membrane over the osteotomy site has been shown to increase the amount of bone formation.

Le Fort I with Bone Graft

The edentulous maxilla resorbs in a superior and posterior direction, resulting in a class III skeletal relationship. For the severely resorbed maxilla, a Le Fort I osteotomy has been shown to be helpful in repositioning the maxilla in an inferior and anterior position, which improves the skeletal relationships (**Fig. 15**).[29–32] Grafting of the created space as well as the floor of the nose is performed. Augmentation of the lateral maxilla is also helpful to regain more width before placing implants. This technique may be more predictable than

attempting to place onlay grafts because of the skeletal mismatch.

Continuity Defects

Large defects involving missing segments of the jaw can present a more challenging defect. Iliac crest bone grafts work very well in conjunction with reconstruction plates (**Fig. 16**).[33] Typically, the defect is treated secondarily from an extraoral approach. If the defect was the result of removal of a malignancy, this will often result in both a hard and a soft tissue defect that may best be treated with free-tissue microvascular flaps. These flaps are more predictable for patients that are undergoing radiotherapy. A disadvantage of these types of flaps is the limited height often gained in trying to rebuild the jaw to form and place dental implants.

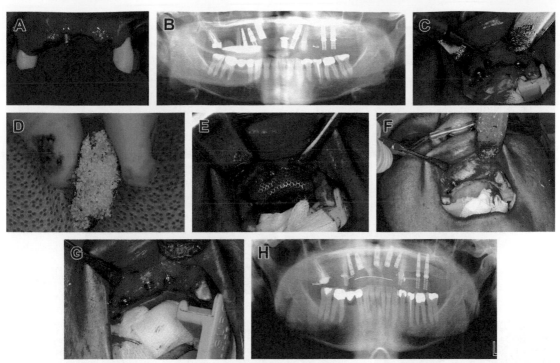

Fig. 13. Maxillary anterior GBR. (*A*) Preoperative with failing implant. (*B*) Radiograph of maxillary defect. (*C*) Removal of dental implant and perforation of cortex. (*D*) Allograft and growth factor mixture placed in titanium mesh. (*E*) Titanium mesh secured in place. (*F*) Titanium mesh removed after healing. (*G*) Implants placed in grafted bone. (*H*) Postoperative radiographs of implants in place.

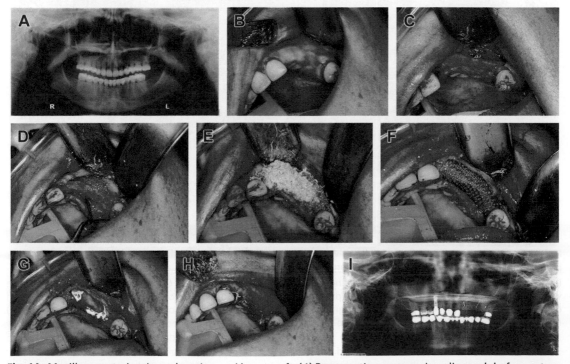

Fig. 14. Maxillary posterior sinus elevation and bone graft. (*A*) Preoperative panoramic radiograph before extractions. (*B*) Maxillary defect. (*C*) Defect exposed including sinus elevation. (*D*) Bone graft and growth factor placed on floor of maxillary sinus. (*E*) Bovine bone and BMP-2 mixture placed laterally. (*F*) Titanium mesh secured in place to contain bone graft. (*G*) Collagen membrane placed over graft. (*H*) Tension-free closure. (*I*) Postoperative panoramic radiograph.

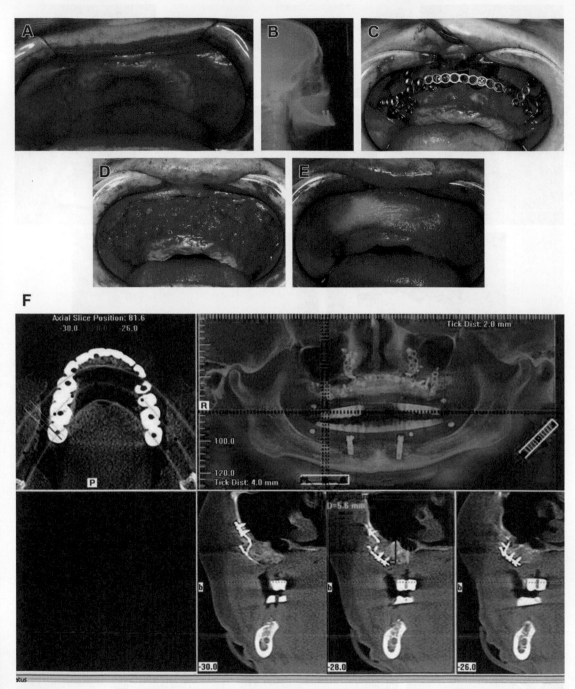

Fig. 15. Maxillary Le Fort I. (*A*) Preoperative view with severe resorption. (*B*) Radiograph of maxillary resorption. (*C*) Le Fort 1 osteotomy. (*D*) Placement of cancellous graft mixed with BMP-2. (*E*) Placement of collagen sponge with BMP over top. (*F*) Radiograph before implant placement. (*G*) Radiographs of anterior region. (*H*) Radiograph of posterior region. (*I*) Postoperative radiograph. (*J*) Uncovering of grafted bone and implant placement. (*K*) Radiograph after implant placement. (*L*) Five-year postoperative occlusion.

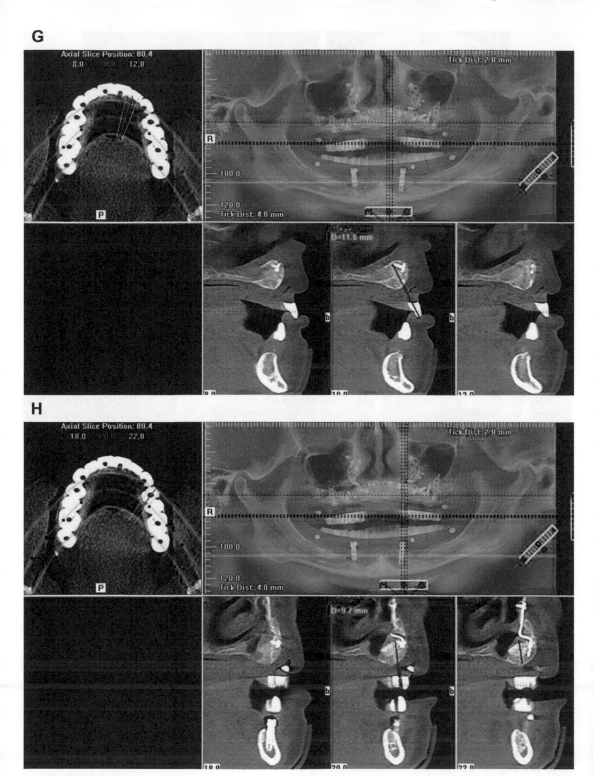

Fig. 15. *(continued)*

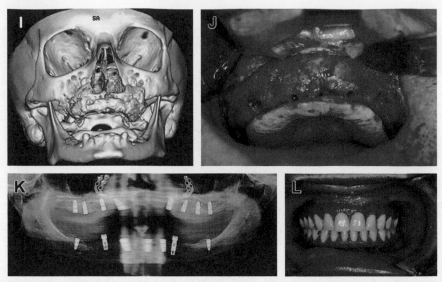

Fig. 15. (*continued*)

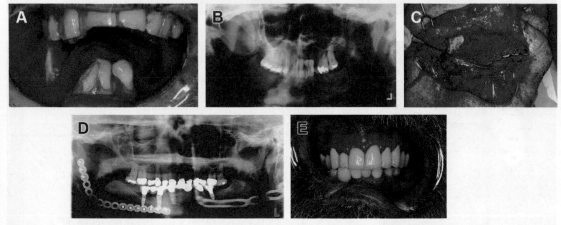

Fig. 16. Mandibular segmental iliac crest bone graft. (*A*) Mandibular segmental defect after resection of tumor. (*B*) Radiograph of mandibular defect. (*C*) Mandibular reconstruction with block grafts covered in cancellous bone. (*D*) Postoperative radiograph with implants in place. (*E*) Restored occlusion.

SUMMARY

Autogenous bone remains the best option for complex defects. The current gold standard for bone grafting is autogenous bone, due to its biocompatibility, lack of antigenicity, osteoconductive, and osteoinducive properties.[2] Additional graft extenders or growth factors may lead to improved outcomes, but more studies are necessary to fully evaluate them and provide an evidence based approach.

REFERENCES

1. Liu J, Kerns DG. Mechanisms of guided bone regeneration: a review. Open Dent J 2014;8:56–65.
2. Duttenhoefer F, Souren C, Menne D, et al. Long-term survival of dental implants placed in the grafted maxillary sinus: systemic review and meta-analysis of treatment modalities. PLoS One 2013;8:e75357.
3. Rocchietta I, Fontana F, Simion M. Clinical outcomes of vertical bone augmentation to enable dental

implant placement: a systematic review. J Clin Periodontol 2008;35:203–15.

4. Wallace SS, Froum SJ. Effect of maxillary sinus augmentation on the survival of endosseous dental implants. A systematic review. Ann Periodontol 2003;8:328–43.

5. Jensen SS, Terheyden H. Bone augmentation procedures in localized defects in the alveolar ridge: clinical results with different bone grafts and bone-substitute materials. Int J Oral Maxillofac Implants 2009;24:218–36.

6. Chiapasco M, Casentini P, Zaniboni M. Bone augmentation procedures in implant dentistry. Int J Oral Maxillofac Implants 2009;24:237–59.

7. Aghaloo TL, Moy PK. Which hard tissue augmentation techniques are the most successful in furnishing bony support for implant placement? Int J Oral Maxillofac Implants 2007;22:49–70.

8. Esposito M, Grusovin MG, Felice P, et al. The efficacy of horizontal and vertical bone augmentation procedures for dental implants - a Cochrane systematic review. Eur J Oral Implantol 2009;2:167–84.

9. Milinkovic I, Cordaro L. Are there specific indications for the different alveolar bone augmentation procedures for implant placement? A systematic review. Int J Oral Maxillofac Surg 2014;43:606–25.

10. Boyne PJ, Herford AS. An algorithm for reconstruction of alveolar defects before implant placement. Oral Maxillofacial Surg Clin N Am 2001;13(3):533–41. Saunders.

11. Avila ED, Filho JS, de Oliveira Ramalho LT, et al. Alveolar ridge augmentation with the perforated and nonperforated bone grafts. J Periodontal Implant Sci 2014;44(1):33–8.

12. Herford AS, Dean JS. Complications in bone grafting. Oral Maxillofacial Surg Clin N Am 2011;23:433–42.

13. Misch CM. Comparison of intraoral donor sites for onlay grafting prior to implant placement. J Periodontal Implant Sci 2014;44:33–8.

14. Herford AS, Stofella E, Tandon R. Reconstruction of mandibular defects using bone morphogenic protein: can growth factors replace the need for autologous bone grafts: a systematic review of the literature. Plast Surg Int 2011;2011:165824.

15. Clementini M, Morlupi A, Agrestini C, et al. Immediate versus delayed positioning of dental implants in guided bone regeneration or onlay graft regenerated areas: a systematic review. Int J Oral Maxillofac Surg 2013;42:643–50.

16. Bell RB, Blakey GH, White RP, et al. Staged reconstruction of the severely atrophic mandible with autogenous bone graft and endosteal implants. J Oral Maxillofac Surg 2002;60:1135.

17. Herford AS. Distraction osteogenesis: a surgical option for restoring missing tissue in the anterior esthetic zone. J Calif Dent Assoc 2005;33:889–95.

18. Elo JA, Herford AS, Boyne PJ. Implant success in distracted bone versus autogenous gone-grafted sites. J Oral Implantol 2009;35:181–4.

19. Herford AS, Tandon R, Stevens TW, et al. Immediate distraction osteogenesis: the sandwich technique in combination with rhBMP-2 for anterior maxillary and mandibular defects. J Craniofac Surg 2013;24:1383–7.

20. Chiapasco M, Romeo E, Casentini P, et al. Alveolar distraction osteogenesis vs vertical guided bone regeneration for the correction of vertically deficient edentulous ridges: a 1-3-year prospective study on humans. Clin Oral Implants Res 2004;15:82–95.

21. Buser D, Ingimarsson S, Dula K, et al. Long-term stability of osseointegrated implants in augmented bone: a 5-year prospective study in partially edentulous patients. Int J Periodontics Restorative Dent 2002;22:109.

22. Von Arx T, Buser D. Horizontal ridge augmentation using autogenous block grafts and the guided bone regeneration technique with collagen membranes: a clinical study with 42 patients. Clin Oral Implants Res 2006;17:359–66.

23. Simion M, Dahlin C, Blair K, et al. Effect of different microstructures of e-PTFE membranes on bone regeneration and soft tissue response: a histologic study in canine mandible. Clin Oral Implants Res 1999;10:73.

24. Chiapasco M, Abati S, Romeo E, et al. Clinical outcome of autogenous bone blocks or guided bone regeneration with e-PTFE membranes for the reconstruction of narrow edentulous ridges. Clin Oral Implants Res 1999;10:278.

25. Von Arx T, Walkamm B, Hardt N. Localized ridge augmentation using a microtitanium mesh: a report on 27 implants followed form 1 to 3 years after functional loading. Clin Oral Implants Res 1998;9:123.

26. Kheur M, Gokhale SG, Sumanth S, et al. Staged ridge splitting technique for horizontal expansion in mandible: a case report. J Oral Implantol 2014;4:479–83.

27. Jensen OT, Bell W, Cottam J. Osteoperiosteal flaps and local osteotomies for alveolar reconstruction. Oral Maxillofacial Surg Clin N Am 2010;22(3):331–46.

28. Jensen OT, Mogyoros R, Owen Z, et al. Island osteoperiosteal flap for alveolar bone reconstruction. J Oral Maxillofac Surg 2010;68(3):539–46.

29. Marchetti C, Felice P, Lizio G, et al. Le Fort I osteotomy with interpositional graft and immediate loading of delayed modified SLActive surface dental implants for rehabilitation of extremely atrophied maxilla: a case report. J Oral Maxillofac Surg 2009;67:1486–94.

30. Chiapasco M, Brusati R, Ronchi P. Le Fort I osteotomy with interpositional bone grafts and delayed oral implants for the rehabilitation of extremely

atrophied maxillae: a 1-9-year clinical follow-up study on humans. Clin Oral Implants Res 2007;18: 74–85.

31. Nocini PF, Bertossi D, Albanese M, et al. Severe maxillary atrophy treatment with Le Fort I, allografts, and implant supported prosthetic rehabilitation. J Craniofac Surg 2011;22:2247–54.

32. Jensen OT, Ringeman JL, Cottam JR, et al. Orthognathic and osteoperiosteal flap augmentation strategies for maxillary dental implant reconstruction. Oral Maxillofacial Surg Clin N Am 2011;23:301–19.

33. Herford AS, Boyne PJ. Reconstruction of mandibular continuity defects with bone morphogenic protein-2 (rhBMP-2). J Oral Maxillofac Surg 2008;66:616–24.

Maxillary Sinus Bone Augmentation Techniques

Vincent Carrao, DDS, MD*, Isabelle DeMatteis, DDS

KEYWORDS

• Maxillary • Sinus • Bone • Augmentation • Implant • Grafting

KEY POINTS

• When faced with implant reconstruction of a maxillary edentulous area with increased pneumatization of the maxillary sinus, treatment planning is of the utmost importance to achieve the desired result.
• The maxillary sinus can be grafted with multiple types of materials; depending on the case, the material of choice should be the one expected to produce the best functional and most stable result.
• Various surgical approaches can be used to achieve optimal results for a graft with enough volume for future implant stability.
• Occasionally the surgeon encounters complications during the surgery or the postoperative phase; the ability to manage these complications is crucial to ensure the best outcome for the patient.

HISTORY OF SINUS LIFTS

• Tatum,[1] 1975: first maxillary sinus augmentation in preparation for dental implant placement
• Boyne and James,[2] 1980: first case report on autogenous grafts for sinus augmentation followed by blade implant placement 6 months after grafting

Anatomy and Physiology of the Maxillary Sinus

The maxillary sinus, also known as the antrum of Highmore, is virtually nonexistent in the neonate. The maxillary sinus pneumatizes over time, thus causing the sinus volume to increase with age. The pneumatization process continues throughout life, resulting in the ever expanding sinus cavity. The bone that is lost secondary to this cavity expansion is the maxillary alveolar bone, which supports the teeth. The maxillary sinus is the largest of the paranasal sinuses. Its function is not well defined; however, it is thought to lighten the skull, humidify inspired air, and contribute to voice resonance.[3]

The sinus is lined with a pseudostratified ciliated columnar/cuboidal epithelium, which is called the schneiderian membrane. This thin membrane produces mucus via goblet cells and contains a basement membrane with occasional osteoblasts. The ciliated membrane functions to transport mucus and debris to the ostium semilunaris, allowing it to exit the sinus cavity. The ostium is situated superior to the depth of the sinus floor therefore requiring the ciliated cells to move the mucus in a cephalad direction. The ostium lies in the semilunar hiatus of the middle meatus of the nasal cavity and is a small opening that can easily be obstructed by mucosal swelling consequently preventing adequate drainage of the maxillary sinus.[4]

Blood supply to the maxillary sinus is robust and derived from the following[3]:

• Infraorbital artery
• Greater palatine artery
• Lesser palatine artery
• Sphenopalatine artery
• Posterior superior alveolar artery

The Mount Sinai Hospital, Mount Sinai Icahn School of Medicine, 1 Gustave L. Levy Place, New York, NY 10029, USA
* Corresponding author.
E-mail addresses: drcarrao@yahoo.com; vincent.carrao@mountsinai.org

Oral Maxillofacial Surg Clin N Am 27 (2015) 245–253
http://dx.doi.org/10.1016/j.coms.2015.01.001
1042-3699/15/$ – see front matter © 2015 Elsevier Inc. All rights reserved.

Diagnosis

As discussed earlier, the pneumatization of the maxillary sinus results in a decrease in alveolar bone height over time, which can present a challenge for practitioners who are asked to reconstruct an edentulous space with the use of dental implants. Maxillary bone tends to have lower density than mandibular bone, which in most cases requires an implant of at least 10 mm or greater to achieve a functional and stable long-term result for the patient requiring dental reconstruction. The basic concept of long-term stability is extremely important when planning for implant placement. An implant that is 10 mm or longer has greater surface area for osseointegration. The axis of rotation is seated deeper into the bone, allowing for greater stability. An implant's surface area can also be increased by the width of the implant. Patients who have had edentulous areas for long periods of time can lose alveolar bone height and width that is not related to pneumatization of the sinus. When alveolar bone height and width are affected by resorption and/or pneumatization, and significant atrophy of the maxillary alveolus has occured, the practitioner is presented with a difficult scenario for reconstruction with dental implants.

When a patient requests maxillary implants, a complete evaluation of the patient must occur in order to arrive at the correct diagnosis and develop a treatment plan that allows for functional and long-term results. The diagnostic process always begins with a complete history taking and physical examination. Taking a good history is vital to surgical success. The age of the patient, medical conditions, medications, past surgeries, and social history ultimately guide the practitioner's decision making and bring to light any issues that may need to be addressed before treating the patient. The following are some common issues that affect treatment related to implant success in the maxilla:

- Immune compromised state
- Bleeding potential
- Delayed and/or poor healing potential
- Other medical comorbidities

Once complete history has been taken, a thorough head and neck examination should be performed. The practitioner can then focus on the maxillary edentulous region to address the patient's chief complaint. When evaluating the edentulous space for possible implant placement, the practitioner needs to take into account the width of the alveolar segment in question from a mesial/distal and buccal/palatal dimension. The mesial/distal dimension should be at least 7 mm

and the buccal/palatal dimension at least 4 mm. One must also take into account bone height of the adjacent teeth if present, occlusal clearance, and the amount of attached gingiva in the edentulous area. The height and width of the maxillary alveolar ridge can be difficult to assess by physical examination alone.

Because the physical examination cannot deliver all the information that is necessary, the next step in the evaluation requires imaging of the area planned for implant reconstruction. At present, 2-dimensional and 3-dimensional (3D) imaging techniques are available. A panoramic radiograph has been the standard for many years for the evaluation of maxillary bone height and sinus floor proximity as it relates to alveolar ridge. There are a few drawbacks with a panoramic radiograph[5,6]:

- It is only 2-dimensional.
- Different magnifications cannot be obtained.
- The soft-tissue image quality is poor.
- Image artifacts are seen.

For these reasons a 3D image has become the image of choice for many practitioners. It gives a much clearer view of the sinus floor, more accurate bone measurement in multiple dimensions, and improved soft-tissue imaging. Most of these 3D images are gathered by office-based computed tomographic scan systems and occasionally from high-resolution hospital/radiology center-based scanners. The advanced 3D image truly helps in the treatment planning of a maxillary implant in close proximity to the maxillary sinus. It provides the practitioner with more accurate information concerning[5,6]

- Height and width
- Sinus floor topography
- Sinus pathology
  - Membrane thickening
  - Air fluid level
  - Presence of a polyp

Once all information is gathered during the workup, the case is planned appropriately and educated decisions regarding implant placement are made. If there is an adequate amount of bone height to accommodate an implant of 10 mm or greater with appropriate width, the practitioner can plan to place an implant in the edentulous area without considering augmentation. If the edentulous area is devoid of adequate bone, an augmentation procedure is necessary. In most cases there is a second practitioner who restores the implant after placement. The plan should be reviewed as a team, being sure to address all the clinical concerns from a prosthetic and surgical standpoint. The treatment plan may involve multiple presurgical visits to fabricate a temporary restoration or possibly a surgical guide. When developing the treatment plan, the practitioner must be sure to inform the patient of all possible treatment options, risks, and complications.

Treatment Planning

On reviewing the gathered information and assessing the patients' needs the surgeon can develop a viable treatment plan. The practitioner may discover that the bone in the edentulous area does not provide an adequate foundation to place implants. The common solution to such a problem is to incorporate bone grafting into the treatment plan. If the surgeon feels there is adequate height of bone but poor buccal/palatal width, the surgeon can avoid grafting the sinus and concentrate on attempting to gain alveolar width with various surgical techniques and materials. If, however, the practitioner is concerned about the height of the alveolar ridge and the proximity of the sinus floor relative to the planned implant placement, a sinus lift procedure needs to be part of the plan to gain alveolar height to place the implants of the appropriate length in the appropriate positions.

A sinus lift procedure refers to a surgical maneuver that elevates the sinus membrane from the floor of the sinus, often including elevation away from the medial and lateral walls. This procedure allows for a graft to be placed inferior to the sinus membrane displacing it superiorly. The lift results in increased height of the alveolar bone once the graft has healed. The success of sinus lifts has been well documented.[7] As the surgeon considers a sinus lift procedure, there are various substances that can be used to graft the floor of the sinus and lift the membrane to achieve the desired bone height. The following are categories of substances that are used to augment the maxillary sinus[8]:

- Xenograft: graft from a different species
- Allograft: graft from the same species
- Autograft: graft from same patient
- Alloplast: graft material that is derived from a nonanimal species, fabricated or engineered

There are many grafting materials available that may be categorized as mentioned earlier. The choice of grafting material for sinus augmentation is determined by a multitude of factors, including the following (**Table 1**)[8]:

- Success rate
- Amount of augmentation required
- Ability to use a donor site
- Cost
- Medical comorbidities

In planning an augmentation, the graft material that has the highest success rate is an autogenous graft. These grafts can be harvested from multiple sites. The donor sites for augmentation are

Table 1
Properties of select graft materials

Graft Material	Origin	Favorable Characteristics	Unfavorable Characteristics
Xenograft	Derived from • Animal bone mineral • Calcifying corals • Calcifying algae	• Limited osteoconductive potential • Biocompatible	
Allograft	Derived from humans • FDBA/DFDBA	• Limited osteoconductive potential • Biocompatible • Faster bone formation (DFDBA)	• Resorption • Prolonged bone formation (FDBA)
Autograft	• Ilium • Tibia • Symphysis • Ramus • Tuberosity	• No disease transmission • Cortical and cancellous (amount varies by site)	• Requires secondary surgical site • Resorption
Alloplast	• Polymers • Calcium phosphates • Bioactive glass • BMP	• Osteogenic, biocompatible • Bonds to bone (bioactive glass) • Osteoinductive (BMP)	• Costly (BMP)

Abbreviations: BMP, bone morphogenic protien; DFDBA, demineralized freeze-dried bone allograft; FDBA, freeze-dried bone allograft.

From Buser D. 20 years of guided bone regeneration in implant dentistry. Hannover Park (IL): Quintessence Publishing; 2009; with permission.

governed by the amount of bone required to achieve the predetermined alveolar height. For large grafts spanning a complete maxillary quadrant that have a minimal amount of native bone, a good source of autogenous bone would be the iliac crest. The greatest amount of bone is harvested from the posterior ilium, with somewhat less from the anterior iliac crest. When sinus alveolar grafting requirements are less substantial, a tibia graft is a good choice as a donor site to provide cancellous bone to achieve the desired height. If the site to be augmented is smaller in nature and autogenous bone is desired, some intraoral sites may also be used to harvest bone (**Fig. 1**)[9,10]:

- Chin
- Ramus
- Tuberosity

If the required amount of grafting material is moderate to small, nonautogenous material is a viable option carrying similar success rates, with a few percentage points less than autogenous grafting. These grafts tend to be the most common types used on patients requiring grafting and implant placement. The following are the reasons for their popular use[9,10]:

- No donor site
  - Decreased postoperative pain and discomfort
- Good success rates
- Easily obtained
- Easy to use

The grafting material used plays a role in the overall outcome and success of the graft in the long term. The success is also multifactorial; the

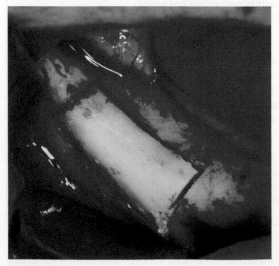

Fig. 1. Ramus graft.

sinus lift procedure lends its success mostly to the actual anatomic site. The schneiderian membrane and maxilla are areas of rich blood supply and osteoblastic activity. The grafted material has a fairly good chance of survival and integration in the maxillary alveolus, producing a new area of bone formation to allow for implant reconstruction. The importance of the membrane in the sinus lift procedure should not be understated. The various techniques used to perform a maxillary sinus augmentation rely on keeping the membrane intact to allow for graft nutrition and a barrier from the maxillary sinus cavity. The surgical technique and surgeon experience are also part of the multifactorial success of sinus augmentation. Choosing the appropriate procedure and applying sound surgical technique in the appropriate surgical site helps in the overall success rate. There are a variety of techniques that are used in various circumstances as discussed later.

Grafting Techniques

Augmentation of the maxillary sinus is a viable option for patients requiring implants placed in the posterior maxillary quadrants who suffer from pneumatization and loss of alveolar bone height.

- Direct technique
  - Two-stage implant placement
  - One-stage implant placement
- Indirect technique
  - One-stage implant placement

The 2 surgical approaches used to elevate the sinus membrane for maxillary sinus grafts are divided into the direct and indirect techniques. The terms apply to the visualization of the schneiderian membrane; if the membrane is identified and lifted under direct visualization, this is considered a direct technique. Conversely, if the procedure being performed did not allow for direct visualization of the membrane being lifted, it is considered an indirect technique. Both the direct and indirect techniques play a role in maxillary sinus augmentation surgery and when used under the right circumstances provide a good long-term stable result with all other factors being equal. The decision to use the direct versus indirect approach for a maxillary sinus lift procedure is governed by the amount of native alveolar bone height present in the edentulous region requiring augmentation. If the height of bone requires more than 3 mm of augmentation, a direct approach should be considered. If the height required is 3 mm or less, an indirect technique can be planned. This reasoning does not prohibit using a direct technique for grafting needs of

3 mm or less; however, the converse is not true. Therefore, planning to use an indirect lift for requirements of maxillary alveolar sites 3 mm or greater may not be the best choice.[9,11]

The direct technique to maxillary sinus augmentation can be as extreme as performed simultaneously with a LeFort I advancement for a severely atrophic edentulous maxilla or can be the more common lateral approach. All the approaches require an osteotomy with identification of the membrane. The osteotomy created should be of adequate size to allow for good visualization and placement of sinus instrumentation and therefore elevation of the sinus membrane (**Fig. 2**).[9]

When dealing with a severely atrophic maxilla that is unable to support a prosthesis, a LeFort I osteotomy with grafting is a viable option. The procedure needs to be performed in the operating room under general anesthesia. A standard LeFort I osteotomy is performed. Once down fractured, the maxillary sinus membrane is elevated and then grafted with cortical cancellous bone from the iliac crest. After augmentation, the maxilla can be advanced if needed according to the preoperative lateral cephalometric analysis (**Fig. 3**).

The lateral approach uses an incision over the midline of the maxillary alveolar crest, incorporating an anterior and posterior vertical release incision. The incision should extend at least 1 tooth past the planned osteotomy on either side, allowing for closure of the flap releases over sound bone. The size of the incision is directly related to the size of the osteotomy, allowing for good visualization and adequate surgical exposure. The osteotomy window is determined by the size of the desired graft and needs to allow for good surgical access to accomplish the planned augmentation.

- Instrumentation
  - Dental hand piece (high speed or low speed)
    - Round or oval bur (diamond or carbide)
    - Specialized side-cutting sinus wall burs
  - Piezoelectric unit
  - Sinus curettes

Once a full-thickness mucoperiosteal flap has been elevated, various bur types are used on a dental drill or a piezoelectric device is used to create an oval or rectangular osteotomy into the lateral maxillary sinus wall, taking care not to perforate through the membrane.

The practitioner has the choice of leaving the center native bone attached to the membrane and elevating the bone to act as roof for the graft or simply removing it. This option is not critical to success and lies in the hands and judgment of the practitioner. The membrane is gently teased from the floor of the sinus and the surrounding walls, producing a pocket to pack the bone of choice for the appropriate situation. The bone graft should provide for at least 12 to 15 mm of bone height. If the site is planned for a 10-mm implant, grafting to a height 2 mm more than needed is advisable to allow for some loss of height during the healing phase. The recommended time for healing is 6 months postgrafting. Once the graft has healed, radiographic imaging is required to evaluate the success of the graft. A panoramic radiograph is adequate for evaluating the final height of the graft as compared with the preoperative radiograph. To obtain a more defined image, a 3D

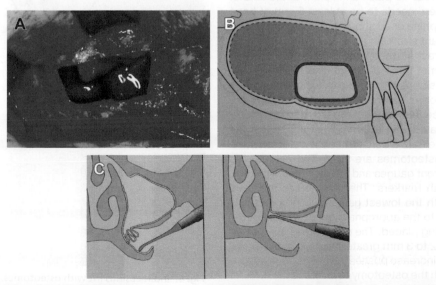

Fig. 2. (*A–C*) Direct lateral window sinus augmentation technique. ([*B, C*] *From* Misch CE. Contemporary implant dentistry. St Louis (MO): Mosby; 1999; with permission.)

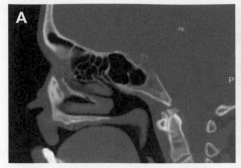
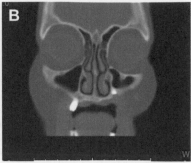

Fig. 3. (*A, B*) Severe atrophy of the maxilla.

scan is preferred, which provides the graft topography width and height. The next phase of treatment is placement of the implant. Placing the implant in a 2-stage format allows the surgeon to place the fixture in the position most suited for the restoration. This technique also lends itself to immediate implant placement. If the native bone height is approximately 5 mm and can provide initial implant stability, the graft and implant are placed simultaneously.[9,12]

The crestal approach is similar to the lateral approach. The difference is the position of the osteotomy, allowing for visualization and elevation of the membrane to pack grafting material. When planning the window over the crest, the incision must be placed appropriately, palatal to the maxillary alveolar crest in the edentulous region. Once a flap is raised, an osteotomy is created with the use of a trephine. The membrane is visualized and lifted. Visualization can be difficult and lifting the membrane challenging. The area can be only grafted or simultaneous implant placement may be considered. To place an implant at the time of grafting, there needs to be at least 5 mm of bone and the trephine used should equate to the appropriate implant size being placed.[12]

The indirect lift technique is a useful approach when minimal bone augmentation is required. A crestal incision is performed to expose the ridge. After incision, small buccal and palatal flaps are raised. Once the ridge is exposed, a small osteotomy is created with a 2-mm twist drill to half the depth of the native bone. After this osteotomy, internal lift osteotomes are used. The osteotomes are of different gauges and are designed with millimeter depth markers. The osteotomes are used starting with the lowest gauge and progressively moving up to the appropriate gauge to accept the implant being placed. The osteotomes are tapped to a depth 2 to 3 mm greater than the native bone. The gauge increase pushes the native bone superiorly through the osteotomy to increase the alveolar height. Because the minimal lift is a blind technique, the membrane is not visualized and thus it is difficult

to identify a tear. Therefore, controlling the depth of the osteotome is important as the bone and membrane are elevated. Once the osteotomy is completed, the implant can be placed safely.[12] An alternate technique is the balloon technique, which is also considered an internal sinus lift technique (**Figs. 4** and **5**).

Complications

When performing surgical procedures, the practitioner always plans for the best outcome. In the best of surgical hands and the best operative environment there is always the possibility of a

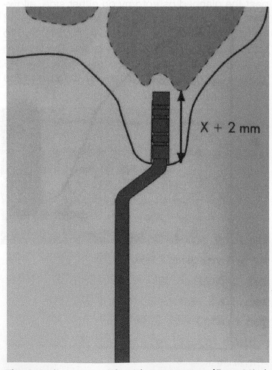

Fig. 4. Indirect sinus lift with osteotomes. (*From* Misch CE. Contemporary implant dentistry. St Louis (MO): Mosby; 1999; with permission.)

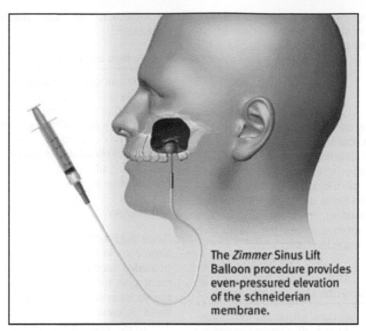

The *Zimmer* Sinus Lift Balloon procedure provides even-pressured elevation of the schneiderian membrane.

Fig. 5. Indirect sinus lift with balloon technique.

complication. A complication can occur during the operative procedure and/or during the postoperative healing phase. Learning to deal with complications when they occur is one of the most important facets of being successful in patient care.

SURGICAL
Membrane Tear/Perforation

Perforations of the schneiderian membrane can occur during sinus augmentation procedures, as the membrane is thin and the topography of the sinus floor is irregular or septated. If a tear occurs, a resorbable membrane is used to repair the defect and allow for a successful sinus augmentation with retention of the graft. Infuse rhBMP has also become an excellent material for the repair of sinus perforations, and it also functions as a bone graft. If the defect is missed or not properly sealed, postoperative imaging may show extravasation of particulate graft into the maxillary sinus, which results in poor graft retention in the area of the desired augmentation. This condition may also predispose to an infection of the maxillary sinus, and close follow-up is indicated. The antibiotic of choice is of the class that covers respiratory flora. If the tear in the membrane is substantial and cannot be corrected with a resorbable membrane or Infuse rhBMP, then the procedure should be aborted (**Figs. 5** and **6**).[11]

Antral Septae

Approximately 20% of maxillary sinuses present with antral septae. These septae may be complete

or incomplete and can complicate sinus augmentation procedures, as it is technically difficult to lift the schneiderian membrane from the septa without a tear. Careful meticulous technique needs to be used to avoid tears. Increasing the size of the access cavity on the lateral wall of the maxillary sinus may be required to allow for complete visualization and augmentation. Preoperative evaluation with radiographic images is a key

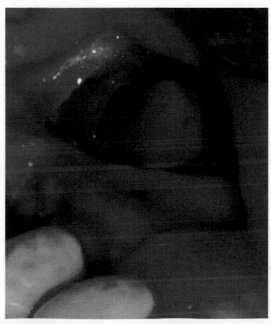

Fig. 6. Tear of schneiderian membrane.

factor in identifying the presence of septae. The radiographs help in surgical decision making, allowing the practitioner to plan where to place the window and what to expect during the procedure (**Fig. 7**).[11]

Bleeding

Significant bleeding can be encountered during sinus augmentation, compromising visibility of the surgical field. This situation can increase the possibility of membrane perforation, which complicates placement of the graft. In the case of severe bleeding, the sinus is packed with packing strips to control bleeding. The planned procedure may need to be aborted unless the bleeding is controlled when the packing is removed.[11]

POSTOPERATIVE CARE
Infection/Acute Sinusitis (3%)

With any surgical procedure, with or without placement of a foreign body or graft, comes the risk for postoperative infection. For acute sinusitis after sinus augmentation, antibiotics covering respiratory flora are indicated. If there is no spontaneous drainage via a developing sinus tract through the incision site, surgical drainage is indicated. Graft failure is expected in these cases. It may also be necessary to remove the grafted material to clear the infection.[9,11]

Nose Blowing

It is imperative to instruct the patient post-op about sinus precautions. Nose blowing with nostrils pinched closed and sneezing with closed mouth needs to be avoided, as this causes increased pressure in the sinuses. After sinus augmentation, the membrane may have areas of weakness or freshly repaired tears. If there is an increase in pressure in the sinus, perforations and

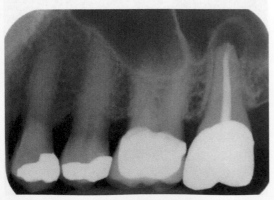

Fig. 7. Septation of pneumatized maxillary sinus.

displacement of the particulate graft are possible.[9,11]

Resorption of Graft

As with any graft material, there is a window in which the graft needs to be stimulated to be maintained and not resorbed. For sinus augmentation, this period is approximately 6 months, after which the graft has undergone solidification and remodeling. If not stimulated in the form of implant placement, the graft continues to resorb and additional grafting may be required.[10]

SUMMARY

Sinus augmentation is a procedure that plays a large role in maxillary implant placement in the posterior maxilla. Arriving at a diagnosis and treatment plan for the augmentation is paramount to the success of the graft and future implant placement. A variety of surgical maneuvers are used. The direct techniques offer the best visualization and control. The indirect techniques are good options when 3 mm or less augmentation is required. The decision to place implants at the time of augmentation should be based on the availability of approximately 5 mm of native bone to produce primary stability. When considering grafting material, autogenous bone has the best chance of success; however, in areas of small grafting demands, or if it is not possible to obtain sufficient autogenous bone, other materials heal well with good success. The use of non-autogenous materials in the office setting will continue to be the main choice for practitioners.

REFERENCES

1. Tatum H Jr. Maxillary and sinus implant reconstructions. Dent Clin North Am 1986;30(2):207–29.
2. Boyne PJ, James RA. Grafting of the maxillary sinus floor with autogenous marrow and bone. J Oral Surg 1980;38(8):613–6.
3. Parks ET. Cone beam computed tomography for the nasal cavity and paranasal sinuses. Dent Clin North Am 2014;58(3):627–51.
4. Bailey BJ. Head and neck surgery – otolaryngology. Philadelphia: Lippincott; 2006.
5. Mora M. Software tools and surgical guides in dental-implant-guided surgery. Dent Clin North Am 2014;58(3):597–626.
6. Guerrero ME. Does cone-beam CT alter treatment plans? Comparison on preoperative implant planning using panoramic versus cone-beam CT images. Imaging Sci Dent 2013;44(2):121–8.
7. Moreno Vazquez JC, Gonzalez de Rivera AS, Gil HS, et al. Complication rate in 200 consecutive sinus lift

procedures: guidelines for prevention and treatment. J Oral Maxillofac Surg 2014;72(5):892–901.

8. Buser D. 20 years of guided bone regeneration in implant dentistry. Hannover Park (IL): Quintessence Publishing; 2009.

9. Tiwana PS. Maxillary sinus augmentation. Dent Clin North Am 2006;50:409–24.

10. Fonseca R. Oral and maxillofacial surgery. St Louis (MO): Saunders; 2009.

11. Misch CE. Contemporary implant dentistry. St Louis (MO): Mosby; 1999.

12. Balaji SM. Direct v/s indirect sinus lift in maxillary dental implants. Ann Maxillofac Surg 2013;3(2): 148–53.

Prosthodontic Considerations in Post-cancer Reconstructions

Piriya Boonsiriphant, DDS[a], Joel A. Hirsch, DDS[b,c],*,
Alex M. Greenberg, DDS[d,e], Eric M. Genden, MD, FACS[f]

KEYWORDS

- Oral oncologic surgery • Biologically driven rehabilitation • Prosthetically driven rehabilitation
- Peri-implant tissue

KEY POINTS

- One of the major challenges facing head and neck oncology is the restoration of function after oncologic surgery of the oral cavity.
- Dental rehabilitation is crucial for achieving good outcomes.
- Presurgical planning with the restoring prosthodontist is mandatory before implant surgery.

The restoration of function after oncologic surgery of the oral cavity constitutes one of the major challenges facing head and neck oncology.[1] For many investigators, the facial skeletal deformities and unfavorable anatomy of the intraoral soft tissues often constituted insurmountable obstacles for dental rehabilitation and functional reconstruction.[2–4] Within the general objective of securing esthetic as well as functional reconstructions, dental rehabilitation is an important consideration for achieving a good outcome. Adequate dental rehabilitation allows the patient to chew food and considerably improves speech and swallowing. Prosthodontic treatments depend on the degree of edentulousness or the type of defect present.

MAXILLARY OBTURATORS

The use of the palatal obturator has been the principal mode of reconstruction of the maxilla after extirpative surgery and is still considered by many to be the gold standard in maxillary reconstruction. The conventional obturator can function quite well as a means of restoring the dentition and separating the oral and nasal cavities. However, many disadvantages of tissue-borne and tooth-borne devices are apparent.

In the partially dentate patient, the obturator is designed to function much like a removable partial denture, with support provided by the remaining palatal bone, the obturated cavity, and the remaining dentition. This situation may lead to unfavorable forces on the remaining dentition, compromising these teeth over time. In more extensive resections, there may be no maxillary bone present to provide obturator support, and, therefore, very few options are available for conventional obturator use.

Endosseous and zygomatic implants can improve a patient's ability to wear these obturators by improving prosthetic stability and retention. In the edentulous patient, use of multiple endosseous implants in the residual alveolar bone can provide a

[a] Advanced Education Program in Prosthodontics, Department of Prosthodontics, College of Dentistry, New York University, 421 First Avenue, New York, NY 10016, USA; [b] Advanced Education Program in Prosthodontics, College of Dentistry, New York University, 421 First Avenue, NY 10016, USA; [c] Private Practice, 570 Park Avenue, NY 10065, USA; [d] Department of Oral and Maxillofacial Surgery, College of Dental Medicine, Columbia University, 630 West 168th Street, NY 10032, USA; [e] Private Practice, 18 East 48th Street, NY 10017, USA; [f] Department of Otolaryngology/Head and Neck Surgery, Mt. Sinai Hospital, 1 Gustave L. Levy Place, NY 10029, USA
* Corresponding author.
E-mail address: jhj90@aol.com

Oral Maxillofacial Surg Clin N Am 27 (2015) 255–263
http://dx.doi.org/10.1016/j.coms.2015.01.007

platform for the fabrication of a retention bar that supports the overlying obturator prosthesis.[5]

RECONSTRUCTED JAWS

The reconstructive surgeon has several options for bony reconstruction of the maxilla or mandible. The specifics of different bone graft harvest sites or free-flap donor sites are beyond the scope of this article. Regardless of the technique used for jaw reconstruction, the surgeon should consider the goal of full dental rehabilitation as the ultimate end point of the reconstruction.

The use of regional flaps and free tissue transfer has allowed for more complex reconstructions and improved functional outcomes. Similarly, the necessity for dental reconstruction has followed with these advancements, and in many cases, it is no longer satisfactory to have a successful cancer ablation and an edentulous reconstructed jaw.

Composite microvascular tissue transfer has revolutionized cancer reconstruction, in that bone and soft tissue can be transferred from a distant site in the same operative encounter as the ablative surgery and, in most instances, from a single donor site. The literature is replete with various donor sites advocated for use in maxillary and mandibular reconstruction, including the ilium, fibula, scapula, radius, rib, and metatarsal. Each donor site has its own advantages and disadvantages, and an ideal replacement for maxillary or mandibular bone and intraoral soft tissue does not exist yet. However, of the donor sites currently available for jaw reconstruction, the ilium and fibula have emerged as the most desirable.[5]

The use of osseointegrated implants in patients with maxillofacial defects has been common practice for the past 15 years.[6] In this sense, Riediger[7] was the first investigator to place deferred implants in microsurgical flaps, and Wei and colleagues[8] helped pioneer immediate implant placement at the time of bone reconstruction.

Presurgical planning with the restoring prosthodontist is mandatory before implant surgery. A surgical guide can be fabricated based on the prosthodontist's estimation of the location of the reconstructed bone and his or her ideal locations for implant fixtures. In some cases, this guide may not be helpful because of inaccurate estimation of the bone location, but can serve as a blueprint for the next-best implant location. Cone-beam computed tomographic scans and implant planning software help mitigate these limitations in the planning phase.[5]

Implants are most commonly placed secondarily into reconstructed jaws, but several investigators advocate implant placement at the time of the initial surgery for reconstruction in cases of benign tumor resections.[9] However, many patients who undergo reconstructive surgery for malignant disease require postoperative radiation therapy. Although the free tissue–reconstructed jaw can withstand radiation therapy quite well, there is no consensus regarding the placement of dental implants before or after radiation therapy. On one hand, if implants are placed secondarily, radiation treatment theoretically predisposes these patients to complications, including implant failure, wound dehiscence, and osteoradionecrosis. Placement of implants at the time of the primary reconstructive surgery also has its potential problems, including the possibility of recurrence of the cancer, interference with radiation treatment, potential for poor implant position, and increased duration of surgery.[5]

The study by Cuesta-Gil and colleagues[10] reported that of the 706 implants used in total, 29 presented with osseointegration failure (global osseointegration failure rate, 4.1%). At the time of dental prosthetic rehabilitation, 31 implants could not be used because of malpositioning (4.4%), in relation to important lack of parallelism and excessive angulation, either lingual or vestibular, or because of placement in posterior sectors with an absence of occlusal space. After prosthetic loading, 52 implants failed (7.4%) in 8 patients. Of these 8 patients, 7 had received radiotherapy. The total failures (osseointegration, malpositioning, and after loading) were 106 implants (global failure rate, 15%).

Implant placement should be prosthodontically driven according to the eventual design of the definitive prosthesis. Collaboration of the restorative and surgical teams is mandatory to confront the esthetic and functional challenges of implant dentistry. The well-established concept of restoration-driven implant placement recommends implant positioning according to prosthetic and esthetic demands to eliminate related complications.[11–13] Digital technology advances have resulted in techniques that can provide optimal 3-dimensional implant positioning with respect to both prosthetic and anatomic parameters.

The predictability and accuracy of maxillofacial reconstruction have progressed rapidly with the advent of virtual surgery. The introduction of computer-aided surgery simulation has enabled surgeons to plan cases virtually and create personalized surgical devices and physical models. This allows the creation of fibula osteotomies that complement the resection exactly.[14] Over the past several years, there has been a trend toward earlier dental rehabilitation as a result of earlier placement of dental implants.[8] The accuracy of computer-aided surgery simulation for fibula reconstruction is now well documented, and this technique has evolved to include immediate dental implant planning and placement.[15,16]

Unfortunately, several anatomic limitations affect the implementation of the prosthetically driven concept, such as the width, height, and angle of the bone. When overlooked, these conditions can lead to unfavorable implant placement, and restoration modifications to counteract implant misalignment are sometimes difficult. Associated complications include off-axis loading.[17] The angled load increases the amount of crestal bone stresses around the implant body, transforms a greater percentage of the force to tensile and shear force, and reduces bone strength in compression and tension.[18] These could lead to interface breakdown, bone resorption, prosthetic screw loosening, and restoration fracture.[18,19] Treatment options to correct severe implant misalignment vary depending on clinical parameters, but usually include the following: (1) implant removal, (2) transformation of the implant into a "sleeper," and (3) restoration with the misaligned implant.[20]

Maxillomandibular tumor ablation frequently results in defects of various tissues, including the lining mucosa, teeth, and bone. In such instances, vascularized tissue flaps that include parts of the extraoral skin can be microtransferred.[21–24] Dental implants are often placed through the grafted skin paddle to restore function and esthetics.[25,26] The nature of peri-implant tissue in implants placed through the skin paddle may differ considerably from that of implants placed through a normal oral mucosa.[21–23] It is generally accepted that a small band of well-keratinized attached gingiva around the implant is necessary for optimal peri-implant soft tissue health and implant longevity. However, implants placed through the skin are surrounded by a thick layer of mobile tissue that may be vulnerable to peri-implantitis. Scientific literature on peri-implant tissue within reconstructed jaws is limited to a few reports and findings, including peri-implant tissue hyperplasia, plaque accumulation, bleeding on probing, and increased pocket depth.[22–24] Studies on longevity of dental implants placed through grafted skin tissue reported varying success rates, from 64% to 100%.[21,25–27]

A major drawback of using skin for the reconstruction of intraoral soft tissues is a hyperplastic/inflammatory response of peri-implant skin and subcutaneous tissues, resulting in the formation of granulomatous tissue that may cause pain and bleeding.[22,28,29] A study by Li and colleagues[30] showed that the implants placed through the skin flaps had significantly higher incidence of peri-implantitis than those placed through the mucosa. Contrary to this finding, those of Kwon and colleagues[24] showed a higher incidence of peri-implantitis around implants placed in mucosa than those in skin tissue, and the researchers concluded that soft tissue origin seemed to have little influence on the development of peri-implant disease. However, Kwon and colleagues[24] also stated that irradiation did not increase the occurrence rate of peri-implantitis.

There is little discussion concerning reactive inflammatory hypertrophy of the skin surrounding the supporting implants. Peri-implant skin health is usually considered a secondary observation affecting some patients and has been reported in clinical case reports focusing on surgical or prosthetic methods to treat the reactive inflammatory tissues.[28,29,31–35] A study by Ahmed and colleagues[36] suggests that inflammatory changes around skin-penetrating oral implants are related to the number of microbial colonies rather than specific pathogens. The skin-penetrating peri-implant tissue is very susceptible to infection; however, the infection process appears to be reversible through the use of effective mechanical oral hygiene at the abutment-skin interface. Therefore, clinicians should consider education and prosthesis designs that promote ease of oral hygiene in this patient population, which often has limitations in oral opening and access to abutments as a result of contracture of the oral vestibule.

A review study by Tang and colleagues[37] reported functional outcomes across 3 categories of prosthetic treatment after microvascular reconstruction of the maxilla and mandible: (1) conventional dental/tissue-supported prosthesis, (2) implant-retained prosthesis, and (3) no prosthesis. Speech outcomes were satisfactory across all groups. Swallowing reports indicated that many patients who received either type of prosthetic rehabilitation resumed a normal diet, whereas those without prosthetic rehabilitation were often restricted to liquid diets or feeding tubes. Patients without prosthetic rehabilitation reportedly had poor masticatory ability, whereas conventional prosthetic treatment allowed some recovery of mastication and implant-retained prosthetic treatment resulted in the most favorable masticatory outcomes. Quality-of-life outcomes were similar across all patients.

The use of a computer-guided approach to implant placement hugely facilitates implant surgery in 3 principal ways.[38] First, implant positions can be planned precisely in relation to the available bone and the planned prosthetic tooth position. Second, the implants can be placed using a flapless, minimally invasive technique through the reconstructive skin flap in the mouth. This was particularly important given the limited time frame available for treatment between healing of the flap and the commencement of radiation therapy and the unfamiliar anatomic environment. Third, implant positioning in this highly complex environment can be planned to avoid the vascular pedicle to the reconstructive bone and skin (damage to this will destroy the free-flap reconstruction completely) and the numerous fixation screws and the bone fixation plate. Dawood and colleagues[38] reported a case on computer-guided surgery for implant placement and dental rehabilitation in a patient undergoing subtotal

Biological Driven Case 1

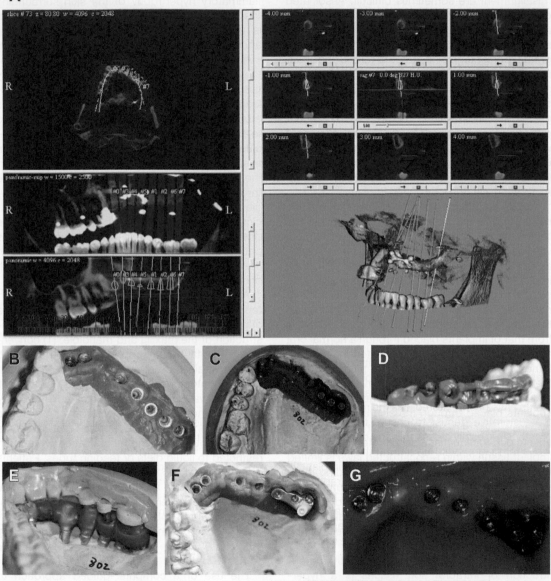

Fig. 1. (A) "Biologically" driven case 1: A patient with history of left hemimaxillectomy with immediate fibular osteomyocutaneous vascularized graft and second-stage placement of dental implants for the treatment of a left maxillary ameloblastoma is shown. Post-reconstruction implant surgical placement was planned on the computer software. (Implant Master, Ident Imaging, New York, NY) Implants were placed according to the plan before surgery. The implant-level impression and the soft tissue final cast were made (B). The verification jig was made on the cast (C) and tried intraorally before the prosthesis fabrication. The framework was waxed up on the final cast (D). The denture teeth were set up on top of the framework wax up on the final cast to verify the available spaces (E). The metal substructure (mesiostructure) was made on the final cast and tried intraorally to correct the angulation of the posterior implants (F, G).

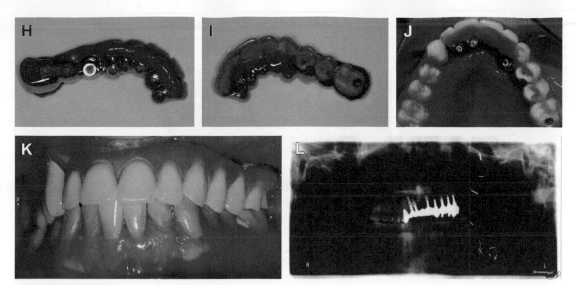

Fig. 1. *(continued)* The design of the substructure overcomes the biologically driven relationship, allowing a proper prosthetic interocclusal relationship. The final prosthesis was made in hybrid design (*H*, *I*). The screw-retained final prosthesis was inserted and evaluated (*J*, *K*). Postoperative panoramic radiograph of dental implant reconstruction (*L*). (*Courtesy of* Surgery: Eric M. Genden, MD, Mount Sinai Hospital, New York, NY; Implant Surgery: Alex M. Greenberg, DDS, New York, NY; Prosthodontics: Joel Hirsch, DDS, New York, NY; Marotta Dental Studio, Farmingdale, NY.)

Biological Driven Case 2

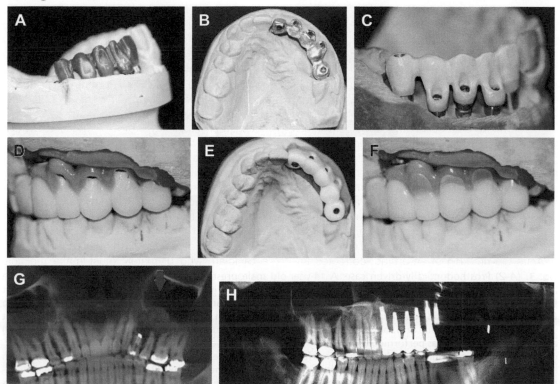

Fig. 2. (*A–F*) "Biologically" driven case 2: A patient with history of left hemimaxillectomy with immediate scapular osteomyocutaneous vascularized graft and second-stage placement of dental implants for the treatment of a left maxillary osteosarcoma is shown. The figure demonstrates prosthetic design modification to overcome the misaligned angulation implants due to limitation of graft design. Indirect pink composite was used to cover the implant access holes and improve esthetics. (*G*) Pre-op CBCT of pathology and (*H*) a post-op Panoramic radiograph of implant Reconstruction. (*Courtesy of* Surgery: Eric M. Genden, MD, Mount Sinai Hospital, New York, NY; Implant Surgery: Alex M. Greenberg, DDS, New York, NY; and Prosthodontics: Joel A. Hirsch, DDS, New York, NY; Marotta Dental Studio, Farmingdale, NY.)

Prosthodontic - Driven Case 3

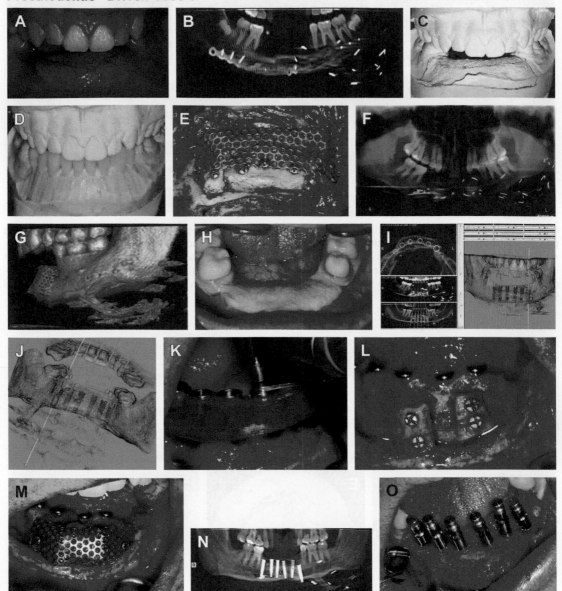

Fig. 3. (*A–Z*) Prosthodontically-driven case: A 14-year-old male presented with history of an initial aggressive anterior segmental mandibular resection for an angiolipoma with immediate free iliac crest block graft that failed at another hospital, and had a secondary fibular osteomyocutaneous vascularized graft (*A, B*). Preparation for diagnostic wax up and debulking of skin graft was performed on the cast before surgery (*C, D*). Subsequent vertical and horizontal bone graft augmentation with recombinant human bone morphogenetic protein (rhBMP) and autogenous bone was performed (*E–G*). Laser hair removal was performed at an earlier visit (*H*). Implant surgical placement was planned on the computer software before surgery (*I–J*). Placement of dental implants with additional horizontal bone graft augmentation with autogenous bone and rhBMP was performed (*K–N*). The implants were uncovered, impressioned, and provisionalized at the same visit after osseointegration of the implants and removal of chin mesh. (*O, P*). The final implant-level impression and final soft tissue cast were made after the soft tissue healed. The intermediate abutment was used at the implant #21 to bring it up to the gingival level (*Q, R*). The cast was scanned. The zirconia substructure was designed and then milled using computer-aided design/computer-aided manufacturing technology (*S–V*). Feldspathic porcelain was veneered to the zirconia framework (*W–Y*). (*Z*) Postoperative panoramic radiograph of dental implant reconstruction. (*Courtesy of* [*A, B*] Surgery: Eric M. Genden, MD, Mount Sinai Hospital, New York, NY; and [*M*] Metronic, Minneapolis, MN; with permission. Alex M. Greenberg, DDS, New York, NY; and Prosthodontics: Joel A. Hirsch, DDS, New York, NY; Franco Petruzziello Dental Lab, New York, NY.)

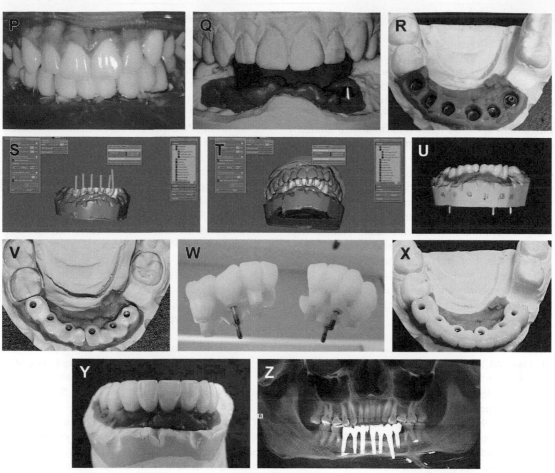

Fig. 3. (*continued*)

Case 4: Peri-Implant Tissue Hypertrophy Case(s)

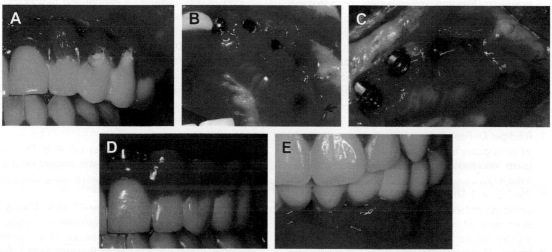

Fig. 4. (*A–D*) Peri-implant tissue hypertrophy and management of granulomatous tissue with blade ablation: peri-implant tissue biologically driven reconstruction following scapular osseocutaneous flap is shown (*A*). Epithelial keratinization is shown by the arrow (*B, C*). Surgical excision of granulomatous tissue was performed. Note composite facial seals over implant access holes due to biologically driven reconstruction (*D*). Peri-implant tissue prosthodontically-driven reconstruction following fibular osseocutaneous flap is shown (*E*). (*Courtesy of* [*A–C*] Surgery: Alex M. Greenberg, DDS, New York, NY; and [*D*] Prosthodontics: Joel A. Hirsch, DDS, New York, NY; Marotta Dental Studio, Farmingdale, NY; and [*E*] Prosthodontics: Joel Hirsch, DDS, New York, NY; Franco Petruzziello Dental Lab, Farmingdale, NY.)

mandibulectomy and microvascular free-flap reconstruction. The dental reconstruction with implant-supported fixed partial dentures took place to the dental scheme–planned preresection, using a computer-guided approach to implant placement in the complex and unfamiliar anatomy of the extensively grafted mandible.

The interdisciplinary team approach with oral surgeons and prosthodontists is guided by cooperation with the oncology surgeons and ear, nose, and throat/plastic specialists to decide whether the dental rehabilitation (reconstruction) will be a biologically or prosthodontic-driven case. Additionally, peri-implant management is demonstrated.

See case 1 (**Fig. 1**) and case 2 (**Fig. 2**) for biologically driven cases, case 3 (**Fig. 3**) for a prosthodontic-driven case, and case 4 (**Fig. 4**) for a Peri-Implant tissue case(s).

REFERENCES

1. Urken ML, Moscoso JF, Lawson W, et al. Systematic approach to functional reconstruction of the oral cavity following partial and total glossectomy. Arch Otolaryngol Head Neck Surg 1994;120:589.
2. Zlotolow IM, Huryn JM, Piro JD, et al. Osseointegrated implants and functional prosthetic rehabilitation in microvascular fibula free flap reconstructed mandibles. Am J Surg 1992;164:677.
3. Komisar A. The functional result of mandibular reconstruction. Laryngoscope 1990;100:364.
4. Urken ML, Buchbinder D, Weinberg H, et al. Functional evaluation following microvascular oromandibular reconstruction of the oral cancer patient: a comparative study of reconstructed and non-reconstructed patients. Laryngoscope 1991;101:935.
5. Kim DD, Ghali GE. Dental implants in oral cancer reconstruction. Dent Clin North Am 2011;55(4):871–82.
6. Parel SM, Bränemark PI, Jansson T. Osseointegration in maxillofacial prosthetics. Part I: intraoral applications. J Prosthet Dent 1986;55:490.
7. Riediger D. Restoration of masticatory function by microsurgically revascularized iliac crest bone grafts using enosseous implants. Plast Reconstr Surg 1988;81:861.
8. Wei FC, et al. Mandibular reconstruction with fibular osteoseptocutaneous free flap and simultaneous placement of osseointegrated dental implants. J Craniofac Sur 1997;8(6):512–21.
9. Chana JS, Chang YM, Wei FC, et al. Segmental mandibulectomy and immediate free fibula osteoseptocutaneous flap reconstruction with endosseous implants: an ideal treatment method for mandibular ameloblastoma. Plast Reconstr Surg 2004;113:80–7.
10. Cuesta-Gil M, Ochandiano Caicoya S, Riba-García F, et al. Oral rehabilitation with osseointegrated implants in oncologic patients. J Oral Maxillofac Surg 2009;67(11):2485–96.
11. Garber DA. The esthetic dental implant: letting restoration be the guide. J Am Dent Assoc 1995; 126:319–25.
12. Smith DE, Zarb GA. Criteria for success of osseointegrated endosseous implants. J Prosthet Dent 1989;62:567–72.
13. de Lange GL. Aesthetic and prosthetic principles for single tooth implant procedures: an overview. Pract Periodontics Aesthet Dent 1995;7:51–61.
14. Levine JP, Bae JS, Soares M, et al. Jaw in a day: total maxillofacial reconstruction using digital technology. Plast Reconstr Surg 2013;131(6): 1386–91.
15. Sharaf B, Levine JP, Hirsch DL, et al. Importance of computer-aided design and manufacturing technology in the multidisciplinary approach to head and neck reconstruction. J Craniofac Surg 2010;21: 1277–80.
16. Roser SM, Ramachandra S, Blair H, et al. The accuracy of virtual surgical planning in free fibula mandibular reconstruction: comparison of planned and final results. J Oral Maxillofac Surg 2010;68: 2824–32.
17. Lewis SG, Llamas D, Avera S. The UCLA abutment: a four-year review. J Prosthet Dent 1992; 67:509–15.
18. Rangert B, Jemt T, Jorneus L. Forces and moments on Branemark implants. Int J Oral Maxillofac Implants 1989;4:241–7.
19. Isidor F. Loss of osteointegration caused by occlusal load of oral implants. A clinical and radiographic study in monkeys. Clin Oral Implants Res 1996;7: 143–52.
20. Lima Verde MA, Morgano SM, Hashem A. Technique to restore unfavorably inclined implants. J Prosthet Dent 1994;71:359–63.
21. Gbara A, Darwich K, Li L, et al. Long-term results of jaw reconstruction with microsurgical fibula grafts and dental implants. J Oral Maxillofac Surg 2007; 65:1005–9.
22. Goiato MC, Takamiya AS, Alves LM, et al. Postsurgical care for rehabilitation with implant-retained extraoral prostheses. J Craniofac Surg 2010;21: 565–7.
23. Chang YM, Coskunfirat OK, Wei FC, et al. Maxillary reconstruction with a fibula osteoseptocutaneous free flap and simultaneous insertion of osseointegrated dental implants. Plast Reconstr Surg 2004; 113:1140–5.
24. Kwon YD, Karbach J, Wagner W, et al. Peri-implant parameters in head and neck reconstruction: influence of extraoral skin or intraoral mucosa. Clin Oral Implants Res 2010;21:316–20.
25. Cheung LK, Leung AC. Dental implants in reconstructed jaws: implant longevity and peri-implant

tissue outcomes. J Oral Maxillofac Surg 2003;61: 1263–74.

26. Raoul G, Ruhin B, Briki S, et al. Microsurgical reconstruction of the jaw with fibular grafts and implants. J Craniofac Surg 2009;20:2105–17.

27. Wu YQ, Huang W, Zhang ZY, et al. Clinical outcome of dental implants placed in fibula-free flaps for orofacial reconstruction. Chin Med J 2008;121:1861–5.

28. Chiapasco M, Biglioli F, Autelitano L, et al. Clinical outcome of dental implants placed in fibula-free flaps used for the reconstruction of maxillo-mandibular defects following ablation for tumors or osteoradionecrosis. Clin Oral Implants Res 2006;17:220–8.

29. Ciocca L, Corinaldesi G, Marchetti C, et al. Gingival hyperplasia around implants in the maxilla and jaw reconstructed by fibula free flap. Int J Oral Maxillofac Surg 2008;37:478–80.

30. Li BH, Byun SH, Kim SM, et al. The clinical outcome of dental implants placed through skin flaps. Otolaryngol Head Neck Surg 2014;151:945–51.

31. Teoh KH, Huryn JM, Patel S, et al. Implant prosthodontic rehabilitation of fibula free-flap reconstructed mandibles: a Memorial Sloan-Kettering Cancer Center review of prognostic factors and implant outcomes. Int J Oral Maxillofac Implants 2005;20: 738–46.

32. Chang YM, Chan CP, Shen YF, et al. Soft tissue management using palatal mucosa around endosteal implants in vascularized composite grafts in the mandible. Int J Oral Maxillofac Surg 1999;28: 341–3.

33. Ueda M, Hata KI, Sumi Y, et al. Peri-implant soft tissue management through use of cultured mucosal epithelium. Oral Surg Oral Med Oral Pathol Oral Radiol Endod 1998;86:393–400.

34. Jaquiery C, Rohner D, Kunz C, et al. Reconstruction of maxillary and mandibular defects using prefabricated microvascular fibular grafts and osseointegrated dental implants—a prospective study. Clin Oral Implants Res 2004;15:598–606.

35. Rohner D, Jaquiery C, Kunz C, et al. Maxillofacial reconstruction with prefabricated osseous free flaps: a 3-year experience with 24 patients. Plast Reconstr Surg 2003;112:748–57.

36. Ahmed A, Chambers MS, Goldschmidt MC, et al. Association between microbial flora and tissue abnormality around dental implants penetrating the skin in reconstructed oral cancer patients. Int J Oral Maxillofac Implants 2012;27(3): 684–94.

37. Tang JA, Rieger JM, Wolfaardt JF. A review of functional outcomes related to prosthetic treatment after maxillary and mandibular reconstruction in patients with head and neck cancer. Int J Prosthodont 2008;21(4):337–54.

38. Dawood A, Tanner S, Hutchison I. Computer guided surgery for implant placement and dental rehabilitation in a patient undergoing sub-total mandibulectomy and microvascular free flap reconstruction. J Oral Implantol 2013;39(4):497–502.

Treatment of the Edentulous Patient

George Shelby White, DDS

KEYWORDS

• Edentulism • Overdentures • Implants • Edentulous population • Quality of life

KEY POINTS

- The edentulous population has been acknowledged as being neglected and denied the opportunity to function at a higher level for decades.
- When considering the quality-of-life issues, the dentally crippled have been hindered from having a more productive life.
- The McGill consensus statement has been the driving force in developing an attitude in dentistry that takes advantage of today's technology.

Edentulism is a chronic debilitating condition that affects millions of peoples' ability to function from a physical and psychological standpoint. No definitive cure exists and, if left unaddressed, the condition will progress. Developing a strategy for treating the edentulous population is essential.[1] The first thing that must be acknowledged is that the edentulous population exists and will continue to increase (**Fig. 1**).

One might conclude that with dental prevention and the advances in dental technology, a decrease in edentulism would occur. According to the statistics of Douglass and colleagues,[2] 33.6 million people needed 1 or 2 dentures in the United States in 1991, and this was predicted to increase to 37.9 million in 2020. The increased longevity of the aged population supports this prediction.

Understanding the role that teeth and alveolar bone play in providing support for a prosthesis to function effectively is important in minimizing the disruptive effects of edentulism. The more effective specialists are in managing these disruptive effects, the more psychologically stable the patient will be. All branches of medicine are addressing quality-of-life issues.[1]

The quality and quantity of supporting anatomic structures contribute to the ultimate success. The results of Tallgren's[3] 7-year studies compare the resorption rate of a complete denture with that of a removable partial denture supported by canines. The studies showed that 6.6 mm of the mandibular process resorbed in patients with complete dentures compared with 0.8 mm in those with removable partial dentures.

The 5-year studies of Crum and Rooney[4] had similar results in their comparison of alveolar bone resorption in patients with complete mandibular dentures versus those with mandibular overdentures supported by canines. They found bone loss to be 5.0 mm in patients with complete dentures compared with 0.6 mm in those with overdentures.

For a denture to meet acceptable functional standards, it must provide support, stability, and retention. With an adequate volume of bone, support and stability can be established. Retention becomes more of a concern with the complete mandibular denture than with the complete maxillary denture.

The American College of Prosthodontists (ACP) developed a diagnostic classification system of complete edentulism based on several factors[5]:

- Bone height of the mandible
- Maxillomandibular relationship

Division of Prosthodontics, Columbia University College of Dental Medicine, 630 West 168th Street, PH 7 East 115, New York, NY 10032, USA
E-mail address: gsw3@cumc.columbia.edu

Oral Maxillofacial Surg Clin N Am 27 (2015) 265–272
http://dx.doi.org/10.1016/j.coms.2015.01.005
1042-3699/15/$ – see front matter

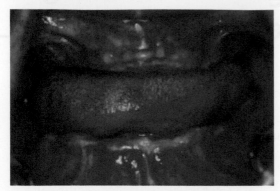

Fig. 1. The forgotten patient with edentulism.

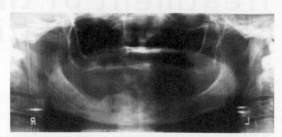

Fig. 3. Pantographic radiograph.

- Residual ridge morphology of the maxilla
- Muscle attachment

Class IV edentulism represents a severely compromised arch that may make treatment extremely difficult. In class IV edentulism, the mandible has a vertical residual ridge height of less than 10 mm (**Figs. 2** and **3**). The maxilla type D is characterized by loss buccal vestibules, hyperplastic or redundant tissue, a palatal vault that does not resist lateral movement, and a prominent nasal spine (**Fig. 4**). These factors indicate a poor prognosis and the need to develop a treatment strategy.[6] The treatment strategy should address both anatomic deficiencies and quality-of-life issues.

Even if the anatomic condition is favorable, it may not meet the expectations or tolerance of the patient with edentulism.

IMPLANT RATIONALE

Patients with edentulism have long been ignored. However, the advent of implants and their acceptance among mainstream treatment options could

affect the manner in which patients with edentulism are treated.[7]

Treatment strategies are multifaceted. A survey was conducted among the faculty of the Columbia University College of Dental Medicine. One question asked was when would the respondent decide to use a 2-implant–supported overdenture; would the respondent fabricate a conventional denture and let the patient decide whether the support of implants was needed, or would the respondent immediately fabricate the 2-implant–supported overdenture? Of the faculty surveyed, 40% elected to wait and let the patient decide whether an overdenture was needed. However, the main consideration one must take into account is complete denture wearers who do not have their dentures remade for at least 6 years; the dentures are not maintained and resorption occurs. The patient with ACP class II edentulism could become ACP class IV, making implant placement more of an issue.[8] Implant placement could have preserved bone for optimum results (**Fig. 5**).

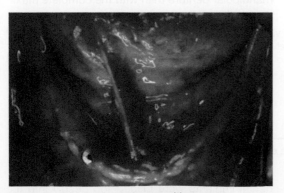

Fig. 2. Occlusal view of the mandibular arch.

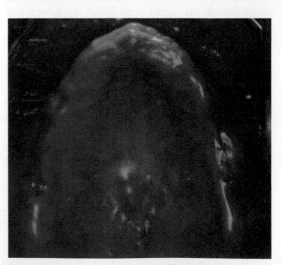

Fig. 4. Occlusal view of the maxillary arch.

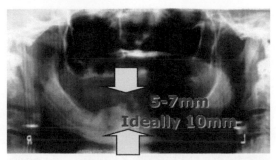

Fig. 5. The window of opportunity is closing to place an implant.

Scientific Support

A panel of experts gathered in Montreal at McGill University to evaluate the best course of action in treating patients with edentulism.[9] The data reviewed from these patients was patient-centered, with quality-of-life issues being the primary consideration. Awad and colleagues[1] compared the patient satisfaction among conventional complete denture wearers versus overdenture wearers. General satisfaction, comfort, and denture stability overwhelmingly favored those with overdentures. The panel concluded that the first choice in restoring the edentulous mandible should be a 2-implant–supported overdenture.[1] The McGill consensus statement has been accepted as the standard of care for the edentulous mandible (see **Fig. 5**).

Adopting the Consensus Statement

The Columbia University College of Dental Medicine decided to adopt the McGill consensus statement into their clinical curriculum. However, an unexpected number of complications occurred that were associated with mandibular overdentures. Incidents occurred in which dentures were not as retentive as expected. More denture fractures were seen. More importantly, patient satisfaction was not as high as expected.

It was therefore necessary to develop a treatment strategy. The first thing that must be recognized is that implant dentistry is a part of mainstream dentistry and should follow the same fundamental principles and requirements. An understanding of bone biology and biomechanics is necessary.

Anatomic landmarks must be evaluated for the role they will play in providing support, stability, and retention for the prosthesis. The buccal shelf provides support to the complete denture because it is a stress-bearing area. A robust posterior ridge provides stability, which resists lateral forces.

Peripheral seal areas provide both stability and retention. On the other hand, the mandibular anterior ridge is not the ideal anatomic area to provide support. The use of implants and their abutments can change the environment of the edentulous ridge.[10] The implant makes the anterior ridge more resistant to ridge resorption and provides stability. The abutment assembly provides retention.

Collaboration with the surgeon is important to ensure proper implant placement. Often there are clinicians who feel that little planning and preparation are involved in implant placement. Ideally, implants should be placed mesial of the canines to avoid tipping (**Fig. 6**). A computed tomography scan verifies that adequate bone is present for the targeted area. A radiographic template should be fabricated from the wax denture using radiographic markers.[8]

Often implants will be found under flanges outside the confines of the denture. Surgical templates can minimize this complication.[11] A surgical template can be converted from the radiographic template (**Fig. 7**); this will prevent an implant from being placed where optimal function will not be achieved (**Figs. 8** and **9**).

Another unfortunate misconception is that taking impressions is not critical to meet all of the standards for overdentures, that the implant will provide all that is necessary.[12–15] However, it is essential that all of the anatomic landmarks be captured in an impression to meet the standards of care (**Fig. 10**).

THE BIOMECHANICS OF THE IMPLANT ATTACHMENT

It may be reasonable to think that the implant attachment should provide stability, support, and retention, but the 2-implant–supported overdenture

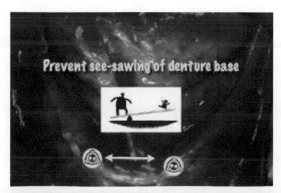

Fig. 6. The attachment should be positioned to avoid denture tipping.

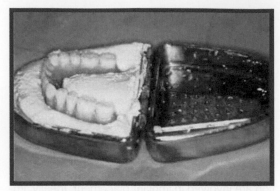

Fig. 7. Duplicator to convert/fabricate into a radiographic or surgical template.

should mainly be used as a source of retention.[16] Using it for support and stability may overload the implant. Only after more implants are used should the overdenture be used for support and stability; this is the rationale for capturing important anatomic areas in the impression. A part of maintaining the mandibular overdenture is accounting for posterior resorption. Resorbing posterior bone places unwanted forces on the 2 implants. It is recommended that the overdenture be relined (see **Fig. 10**).

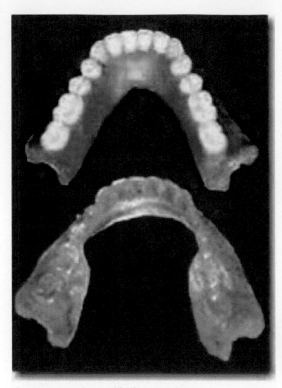

Fig. 9. Surgical mandibular template.

Studs Versus Bar

Traditionally, bar attachments have served as a preferred option in the support on both natural teeth and implants for overdentures. The McGill consensus statement stated only 2% of the edentulous population used implants. The assumption was that cost played a role in this low rate. The bar attachment was costly, whereas stud types (O-rings or Locator attachments) provide a reduced cost that is more affordable to the patient population. Columbia University College of Dental Medicine selected the Locator by Zest as the

preferred attachment because of its limited vertical space, easy maintenance, and effective retentive elements. The assembly requires 3.17 mm of vertical height and can correct 40° of deviation (**Fig. 11**). It has been suggested that the use of a bar should be considered in patients with extreme angulation between 2 or more implants.

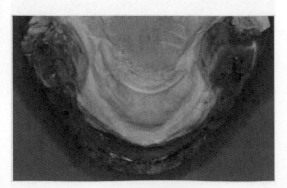

Fig. 8. Surgical mandibular template.

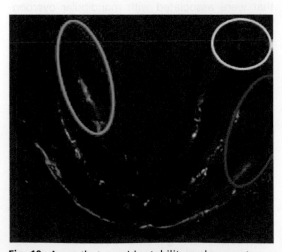

Fig. 10. Areas that provide stability and support.

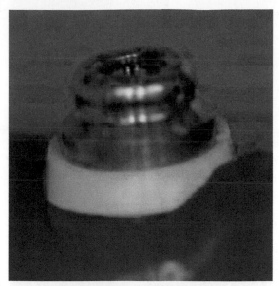

Fig. 11. Locator abutment with space.

TWO-IMPLANT–SUPPORTED OVERDENTURE

The 2-implant–supported overdenture procedure has become an option well suited to be taught at a predoctoral level.[17] It is an ideal entry-level procedure that illustrates how implantology is a part of the mainstream of dentistry (**Fig. 12**).

The Locator attachment has been ideal for the overdenture, if the implant has been placed in the correct location (**Fig. 13**). A checklist of proper protocol is as follows:

- Have the patient wear the denture before the attachments are inserted to allow time to adjust occlusion and relieve sore spots.
- Ensure that the convergence angle is within the 40° limit. A retention male is also available

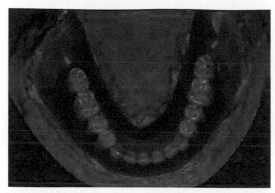

Fig. 13. The wax-up with implant and housing located directly under the mesial of the canine.

for extended ranges. If the angle is excessive, a bar may be considered.
- Evaluate for the need for metal support in the denture base (**Fig. 14**).
- Measure the soft tissue sulcus from the platform of the implant. The measurement should be recorded 1 to 2 mm above the crest of soft tissue (**Fig. 15**).
- The abutment and housing should be within the confines of the denture directly under the denture teeth and slightly lingual. It should be slightly mesial to the canine to avoid seesawing or tipping (**Figs. 16** and **17**).
- An accepted option is to self-cure the attachments in the denture base right at chairside. The denture should be relieved to accommodate the Locator housing. Care should be taken to confirm that the area is relieved adequately for the metal housing. The housing should not bind and must have adequate room for the self-curing material.

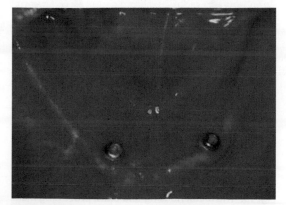

Fig. 12. Locator abutment (occlusal view). (*Courtesy of* Dr Nurit Bittner, New York, New York.)

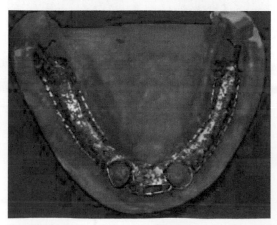

Fig. 14. A metal reinforcing frame is used to avoid fracture. (*Courtesy of* Dr Nurit Bittner, New York, New York.)

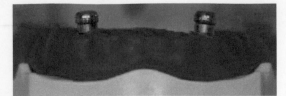

Fig. 15. Locator with metal housing. (*Courtesy of* Dr Candice Zemnick, New York, New York.)

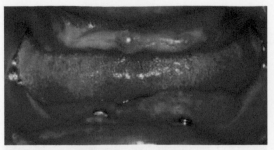

Fig. 17. Locator abutment (frontal view). (*Courtesy of* Dr Nurit Bittner, New York, New York.)

- After the abutment is properly inserted, check to make sure the soft tissue is at the right height (1–2 mm over the soft tissue crest).
- Place the relief spacer and the housing with processing element on the abutment (see **Figs. 11** and **16**).
- Insert the denture, ensuring that it does not bind with the housing.
- Add self-curing acrylic into the relieved area, taking care to avoid overfilling to prevent the denture from locking onto the implant.
- After the acrylic has set, remove the denture from the mouth. Remove excess material, especially around the lips of the metal housing (**Figs. 18** and **19**).
- Remove the black processing male and replace it with the appropriate retention male, which meets the selected strength (**Fig. 20**).
- The denture can be reinserted to evaluated and make adjustments.

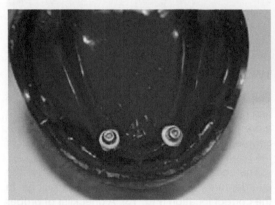

Fig. 18. Locator abutment, housing, and spacer. (*Courtesy of* Dr Candice Zemnick, New York, New York.)

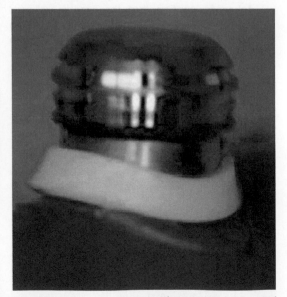

Fig. 16. Locator abutment with metal housing and spacer. (*Courtesy of* Dr Candice Zemnick, New York, New York.)

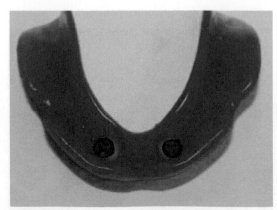

Fig. 19. The metal housing and black processing male. (*Courtesy of* Dr Candice Zemnick, New York, New York.)

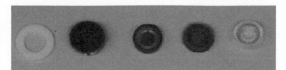

Fig. 20. The metal housing, spacer, and retention males.

- Instructions to insert and remove the denture should be given to the patient (**Fig. 21**).
- Home care instructions should be provided before the patient leaves wearing the prosthesis.
- The postoperative visit is similar to that for a conventional complete denture or removable partial denture. The patient may need sore spots relieved and the occlusion adjusted. The most common concern is removing the prosthesis.

THE BAR-SUPPORTED OVERDENTURE

The bar-supported overdenture has been the choice of many clinicians for decades. With the development of the newer stud-like attachments (Locator), many clinicians have moved away from using them because of costs.[7]

Stud-like attachments come with their share of concerns. The Locator has angulation limitations. With the maxillary overdenture, 4 implants are suggested. Getting these implants to meet the angles of tolerance suggested by the companies is not possible. The bar can accommodate extreme

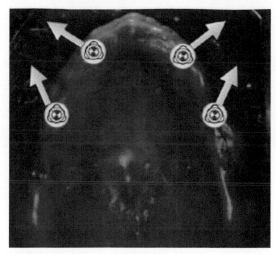

Fig. 22. Multiple implants with angles that pose problems for Locator attachments.

angle deviation. Hader bars with clips are commonly used. Care should be taken to ensure adequate interocclusal space is available (**Figs. 22** and **23**).

The implant abutment is designed to provide retention. The vertical and lateral forces generated by the prosthesis may overload the implant; the bar manages these types of forces. Data show that the 19% failure rate of implants is associated with maxillary overdentures.[18,19] Providing at least 4 maxillary implants, joined with a bar for support, could better accommodate the forces generated by the maxillary overdenture.

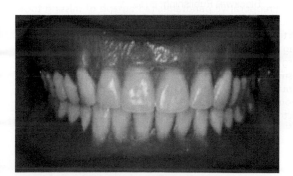

Fig. 21. A conventional maxillary complete denture opposes a mandibular 2-implant–supported overdenture. (*Courtesy of* Dr Nurit Bittner, New York, New York.)

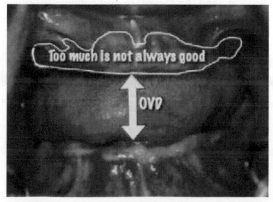

Fig. 23. Excessive amounts of maxillary alveolar bone could restrict the use of clip bars to support the maxillary overdenture. Removal of bone to provide interocclusal space may be indicated.

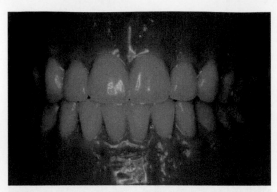

Fig. 24. A mandibular 2-implant–supported overdenture opposing a conventional maxillary complete denture. The patient with edentulism assumes higher standards for better function, esthetics, and quality of life.

SUMMARY

The edentulous population has been acknowledged as being neglected and denied the opportunity to function at a higher level for decades. When considering the quality-of-life issues, the dentally crippled have been hindered from having a more productive life. The McGill consensus statement has been the driving force in developing an attitude in dentistry that takes advantage of today's technology.

The overdenture has proven to be effective in meeting the needs of the edentulous population. However, with the rate of use at only 2%, more must be done to increase its adoption.

Appropriate care now reaches those who would have been overlooked. Implants have been used to serve not only the affluent but also those less fortunate. A generation of dentists is being trained who will accept their moral obligation to treat those in need. As Douglass and colleagues[2] point out, the edentulous population exists and will continue to increase.

Technology will continue to advance and patients with edentulism should never be forgotten and excluded from future planning **(Fig. 24)**.

REFERENCES

1. Feine J. Implant overdentures: the standard of care for edentulous patients. Carlsson (GA): Quintessence Publishing Company; 2003.
2. Douglass CW, Shih A, Ostry L. Will there be a need for complete dentures in the United States in 2020? J Prosthet Dent 2002;87:5–7.
3. Tallgren A. The continuing reduction of residual alveolar ridges in complete denture wearers: a mixed-longitudinal study covering 25 years. 1972. J Prosthet Dent 2003;89:427–35.
4. Crum RJ, Rooney GE Jr. Alveolar bone loss in overdentures: a 5-year study. J Prosthet Dent 1978;40:610–3.
5. McGarry TJ, Nimmo A, Skiba JF, et al. Classification system for the completely dentate patient. American College of Prosthodontics. J Prosthodont 2004;13(2):73–82.
6. McGarry TJ, Nimmo A, Skiba JF, et al. Classification system for complete edentulism. Dent Today 2001;20(10):90–5.
7. Felton DA. Edentulism and comorbid factors. J Prosthet Dent 2009;18:88–96.
8. Laney W, Salinas T, Carr AB, et al. Diagnosis and treatment in prosthodontics. Chicago: Quuintessence Publishing Company; 2011.
9. Morrow R. Tooth supported dentures part II. J Prosthet Dent 1969;22:414.
10. Krol A, Jacobson T, Finzen F. Removable partial denture design. San Francisco (CA): Indent; 1999.
11. Misch C. Dental implant prosthetics. St. Louis (MO): Mosby; 2005.
12. Morrow R, Feldmann EE, Rudd KD. Tooth-supported complete dentures: an approach to preventive prosthodontics. J Prosthet Dent 1969;21:513–22.
13. Marrow R, Rudd K, Rhoads J. Dental laboratory procedures, complete dentures. St. Louis (MO): Mosby; 1980.
14. Preiskel HW. Overdentures made simple. Chicago (IL): Quintessence Publishing; 1996.
15. Miller PA. Complete dentures supported by natural teeth. J Prosthet Dent 1958.
16. Froum S. Dental implant complications: etiology, prevention, and treatment. West Sussex (UK): Wiley-Blackwell Publishing; 2010.
17. Sadowsky SJ. Mandibular implant-retained overdentures: a literature review. J Prosthet Dent 2001;86:468–73.
18. Goodacre CJ, Bernal G, Rungcharassaeng K, et al. Clinical complications in fixed prosthodontics. J Prosthet Dent 2009.
19. Goodacre CJ, Bernal G, Rungcharassaeng K, et al. Clinical complications with implants and implant prostheses. J Prosthet Dent 2003;90(2):121–32.

Dental Extraction, Immediate Placement of Dental Implants, and Immediate Function

Ole T. Jensen, DDS, MS

KEYWORDS

• Dental extraction • Dental implants • Immediate placement • Immediate function

KEY POINTS

• Immediate function requires adequate implant stability.
• Immediate function requires prosthetic stability, particularly when multiple implants are loaded.
• Factors to consider for immediate implants into extraction sites are thickness of socket walls, thickness of gingival drape, optimal position of the implant, and patient factors such as hygiene and smoking cessation.

The placement of implants into a traumatic osseous wound in which the pattern of postextraction healing is epigenetically and biomechanically determined suggests caution on the part of dentists and patients desiring immediate function treatment.[1] What happens after extraction is patterned in the biology and cannot be substantially changed at baseline by any effort to replace teeth immediately with implants. Therefore, treatment must be compensatory, that is, treatment must include conjunctive augmentation procedures, often both hard and soft tissue, to account for loss of postextraction volume.[2–4] The art of treatment, even guesswork, of what should be done is a clinical challenge because inevitably postextraction bone loss is indeterminate.

A recent review of immediate placement of single-tooth implants by Vignoletti and Sanz[5] concluded that immediate placement, even with grafting procedures, is still not fully validated with no clear evidence of consistent clinical outcomes. One of the reasons for this is reports are mostly based on implant persistence. Findings in the literature are usually 2 years or less with descriptive findings most often emphasized. Quantitative findings, particularly in the esthetic zone, are difficult to determine because adjacent teeth and supporting bone can mask relative peri-implant failure. Even in longer-term studies, such as a 9-year study done by Buser and colleagues,[6] there was found to be about a 5% incidence of complete resorption of the facial bone graft. When adjacent implant cases are reported or multiple extraction sites are addressed, there is much less information regarding gingiva-esthetic and/or osseous stability around immediate placement implants. If one reads the literature critically, a bias for reporting successful outcomes is obvious. In other words, clinicians seldom report treatment failures.[7,8]

Figs. 1 and **2** show a 6-month treatment sequence of periapical radiographs of complete maxillary arch implant treatment. The 60-year-old female patient was a healthy nonsmoker in which extractions, implant placement, and peri-implant bone grafting were done uneventfully as was placement of the provisional restoration, all completed on the same day. By month 3, one central incisor implant became infected (number 9) and was treated by antibiotics only. By month 4, it was decided to remove the implant due to

School of Dentistry, University of Utah, 530 South Wakara Way, Salt Lake City, UT 84108, USA
E-mail address: ojensen@clearchoice.com

Oral Maxillofacial Surg Clin N Am 27 (2015) 273–282
http://dx.doi.org/10.1016/j.coms.2015.01.008
1042-3699/15/$ – see front matter © 2015 Elsevier Inc. All rights reserved.

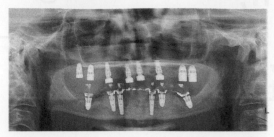

Fig. 1. Complete extraction of the maxillary dentition was followed by placement of 8 dental implants placed vertically into extraction sockets, all of which had insertion torque values greater than 50 Ncm and were immediately loaded on the same day.

3 mm of crestal bone loss despite the implant being firmly integrated apically (**Fig. 3**). A flap of the anterior arch revealed generalized crestal bone loss and compromised osseointegration of 3 other anterior implants necessitating removal and replacement of all 4 implants (numbers 5, 8, 9, and 12). Why did this happen? Can this be attributed to technical factors or armamentarium? Or is it strictly an effect of underlying biology?

The initial postplacement computerized axial tomographic scan showed well-grafted implants, all of which had insertion torques greater than 50 Ncm with implants placed deep into the extraction sockets (about 4 mm). Grafting material was composed of 50% by volume of an allograft/bone morphogenic protein-2 admixture. The prosthesis had never become loose or unstable. Following removal of the 4 implants, it was noted that facial bone had remodeled extensively around the arch. There was reductive vertical and horizontal bone loss of 2 to 3 mm throughout. Re-treatment implants were placed into adjacent sites or left submerged. The follow-up provisional required modification to make up for significant loss of facial bone support. One had the sense that remodeling events could not be curtailed despite efforts to prevent them.

A review of the initial surgery after extraction revealed very thin facial plates of bone with relatively

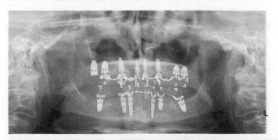

Fig. 2. A screw-retained cross-arch stabilized interim prosthesis is placed on the day of surgery. The prosthesis is made with emergence profile principles based on single-tooth implant restorations.

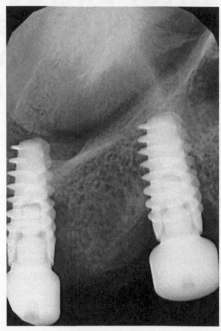

Fig. 3. Four months after immediately loading, there is bone loss evident around the anterior implants. A mucoperiosteal flap is raised to inspect the sites and a decision is made to remove the 4 anterior implants due to generalized bone loss despite continued implant stability.

thin interseptal bone between extraction sites (**Fig. 4**). In addition, there was reduced alveolar height overall, suggestive of short face syndrome such that implant lengths were generally short (**Fig. 5**). Overall, there was reduced bone mass. Although implants were well spaced apart and implants placed well away from the facial plate with intervening grafting material, failure still occurred. The important factors favorable for implant success mentioned by Vignoletti and Sanz include the following:

1. Substantial thickness and integrity of socket walls
2. Adequate vertical and horizontal position of the implant
3. Gingival thickness and integrity
4. Patient factors such as hygiene and smoking

Of these factors, the existing bone volume and its capacity to heal are most important. When there is not enough bone to support implants or bone structure resorbs away, implant failure occurs even in the setting of multiple splinted implants as was found in this example patient.

This implant failure is further exemplified in looking at cases in which multiple implants are lost, so-called cluster failures. Jempt and Hager[7] found in a review of 17 cluster-failure patients that the

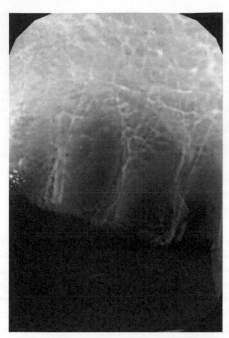

Fig. 4. The original extraction site shows thin interseptal bone in a "short face" alveolus, indicating a relative deficiency in osseous structure necessary for stable immediate function with dental implants.

most important factor was deficiency in supporting bone. Their study concerned delayed placement implants and delayed loading of axially placed implants. What about the more demanding setting of dental extractions and immediate placement? For immediate function, instead of osseointegration, there is a need for mechanical fixation initially, which, if not present, can lead to implant mobility, bone loss, and failure. Therefore, the possibility of mechanical failure from immediate loading bone stress prior to osseointegration

becomes an important complicating factor to consider.

Publications regarding extraction site implant placement are almost all exclusively single-tooth sites with complete arch treatment extrapolated from this data.[9,10] One thing to consider for reducing the risk of multiple extraction site instability in the immediate load case is to reduce alveolar height and place a fixed denture prosthesis such as is done in all-on-4 therapy; this very much reduces the risk for alveolar bone instability around implants. The all-on-4 generally requires about a 5-mm vertical reduction in bone height, creating a level plane termed the all-on-4 bone shelf.[11] The use of the bone shelf has led to very stable findings over time. In other words, implants are placed into sites in which the bone walls surrounding the implants are thick and socket bone grafting is unnecessary.

An example of a maxillary bone shelf is shown in **Fig. 6**. Panoramic radiographs of different patients, a maxillary treatment after 2 years (**Fig. 7**), and a mandibular treatment after 4 years (**Fig. 8**) show very stable bone despite removal of multiple infected teeth, osseous leveling, and implant placement done on the same day.

This approach has been shown to be more stable than the multiple extraction implant case over time and with substantially much less risk for the patient. If an implant is lost in the all-on-4 scheme, it can easily be replaced and at low cost without additional bone grafting. This is not the case with multiple implant treatment, which is generally more invasive and requires bone grafting and considerable re-treatment cost. Multiple tooth reconstructions are prohibitive for several reasons

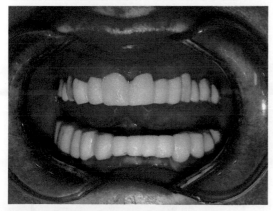

Fig. 5. Following the placement of 8 implants into extraction sites, an emergence profile screw-retained temporary bridge was placed on the same day as surgery.

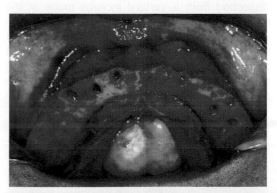

Fig. 6. The all-on-4 bone shelf serves several functions, including providing for adequate restorative space. Shown here is a maxillary bone shelf after a 5-mm reduction. Optimal bone support areas for implants are easily selected to improve chances for immediate function as well as to avoid bone grafting or placement into sites that may undergo reductive remodeling.

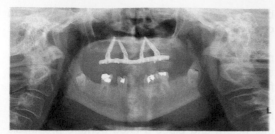

Fig. 7. A maxillary all-on-4 final restoration, now 2 years in function, with stable bone levels around the implants consistent with a stable all-on-4 shelf.

even though the technique is well based on the single-tooth immediate extraction/implants placement model.

Single-tooth extraction and immediate replacement with same-day implant-supported provisionalization is well founded and is considered optimal treatment for loss of nearly all single teeth in the anterior maxilla. An example of how immediate load single implants in the esthetic zone should be done, as shown in **Figs. 9–16**. Following extraction of a central incisor tooth, the socket is found to be ovoid with a very thin facial plate of bone. The implant is placed toward the palatal wall, leaving a 2-mm gap between it and the 1-mm residual facial place, about 3 mm overall. Because part of the blood supply of the facial plate is from the periodontal ligament (PDL), facial plates that are 1 mm or less can be expected to resorb away necessitating both hard tissue and soft tissue grafting.[12] Xenograft is probably the best material to place in the socket gap to avoid late-term resorption.[13] In anticipation of resorption of the facial plate, a connective tissue graft is placed facially using a split-thickness soft tissue flap to create a pocket dissecting from a vertical incision made at the maxillary frenum. The graft is sutured into position with resorbable suture. The angle of the implant should be through the incisal edge. The implant body should not be beyond the buccal line.[14] Apical fixation of the implant into the nasal floor is done to increase insertion torque. Greater than

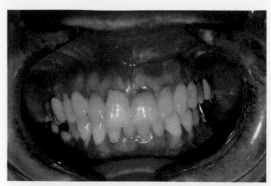

Fig. 9. A patient presents with internal resorption of a left maxillary central incisor.

30 Ncm is desirable.[15] Six millimeters of circumferential bone is minimally needed to insure enough bone for maintenance of mechanical fixation until osseointegration can occur.[16] The patient after 1 year appears to have a stable outcome within bone and soft tissue despite the dynamic nature of dental root replacement with an orthopedic bone screw (**Fig. 17**).

When multiple extraction sites are treated with implants, it is advisable to alternate implants such that 6 or 8 implants are used to treat an entire arch. However, locations such as between the first molars and second premolars and sometimes central incisors can sometimes have less than 4 mm of bone between implants, increasing the risk for bone resorption due to implant proximity.

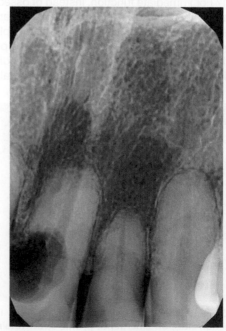

Fig. 10. Radiographic presentation shows internal resorption of tooth root.

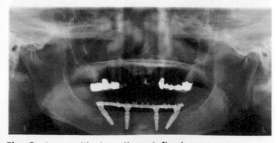

Fig. 8. A mandibular all-on-4 final restoration, now 4 years in function, with stable bone levels around the implants consistent with a stable all-on-4 shelf.

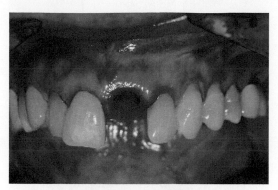

Fig. 11. After extraction gingival findings. There is an intact but thin facial plate present.

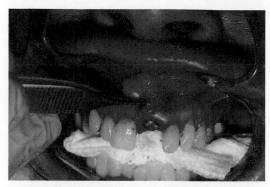

Fig. 13. Following grafting of the implant to facial plate gap with xenograft, a connective tissue graft is placed through a frenal incision into a supraperiosteal pocket is prepared in front of the implant site.

Therefore, implants can be placed in a pattern of first molars, second premolars, canines, and centrals, leaving a well-distributed implant scheme. For 6 implants, the first molars, first premolars, and lateral incisor locations may be optimal. For a 4-implant scheme, implants are placed about 20 mm apart with first molar and just anterior to the canine positions optimal.

All-on-4 treatment is typically an immediate loading situation.[17] The arch may have been previously edentulated or may sometimes be edentulated at the time of implant placement. In either case, the bone is leveled and interocclusal space is increased as needed to provide room for the fixed denture prosthesis. This space is approximately 15 mm per arch.[18] Therefore, if both arches are done, the interarch distance should be 30 mm. This distance is required to have enough room for dental abutments, the titanium bar, and the prosthesis itself. If zirconium is used, bone reduction must be sufficient to provide adequate thickness to maintain zirconium integrity.

The foundation of the all-on-4 is the all-on-4 bone shelf. The bone shelf provides multiple advantages to the surgeon besides establishing prosthetic guidelines, which include visualization

of optimal implant sites, removal of diseased bone, reduction of extraction sites, better visualization of the nerve and sinus anatomy, better visualization of undercuts, and improved access to basal bone for apical engagement of implants.[11,18] In addition, the surgeon is able to better visualize the distribution of implants, implant angles, and abutments angles. The surgeon should place angle-correcting abutments before flap closure. This angle-correcting abutment ensures there is no bone interference of abutment seating, which can be observed by direct vision in the presence of the shelf. Abutment position is then verified radiographically.

One of the important aspects of the shelf is the ability to better conceptualize and visualize angled implant placement. Implants are commonly placed at 30° angles best related to a horizontal plane, such as the bone shelf, enabling implant placement to avoid the nerve in the mandible, and the maxillary sinus and nasal cavities. For the maxilla, an M-shaped pattern of implant placement is achieved by 30° implant insertion, which avoids all pnuematization (**Fig. 18**).[19,20] For the mandible, the posterior implants are usually angled at 30° to avoid the mandibular nerve, which is done by

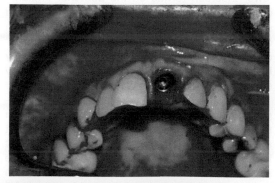

Fig. 12. The implant is placed against the palatal wall and about 2 or 3 mm away from the buccal wall.

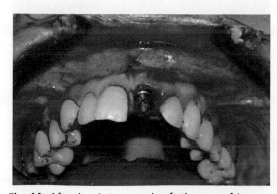

Fig. 14. After hard tissue and soft tissue grafting.

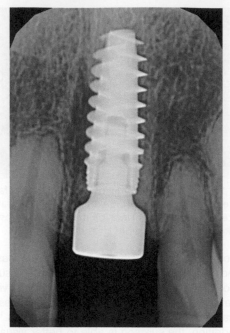

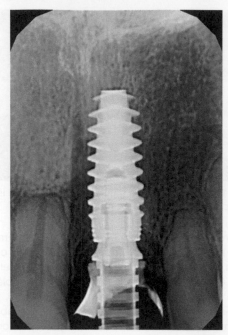

Fig. 15. Radiographic appearance on the day of implant placement.

Fig. 17. One year after treatment, a periapical radiograph reveals a well-integrated fixture with stable bone levels.

angling the implants a few millimeters in front of the foramen (**Fig. 19**). Depending on how much bone is between the shelf and the foramen, implants can actually be placed posterior to the nerve.[21]

Avoidance of vital structures, increased bone stability, and reduced need for bone grafting are commonly represented as the most important advantages of implant angulation. However, there has not been enough wholesale acceptance of the technique. However, these are not the main advantages of implant angulation. The main advantage is biomechanics. Implants inserted apically into available cortical bone, particularly in the maxilla, enable immediate functional

loading. It is impossible to gain fixed implants axially as often as can be done using off-axis.

The importance of angulation is access to cortical bone such as at the lateral pyriform rim. This bone provides increased insertion torque. Insertion torque has been determined to directly correlate to bone density as well as bone to implant contact.[22,23] Minimum insertion torque has not been established, but as a general rule for 4 implants to be immediately loaded, there should be a minimum of 30 Ncm per implant or 120 Ncm *composite* insertion torque.[24] If 1 or 2 implants are less than 30 Ncm, other implants must be more than 30 Ncm to maintain the 120 Ncm minimum. In the maxilla, it is most important for the anterior implants to be well fixed. Therefore, lower insertion torque on the posterior implants can be acceptable in a cross-arch splinted scheme provided there is compensation from other loaded implants.[20] Patients who brux, particularly if opposing natural dentition is present, may loosen immediately loaded implants even if they exceed 200 Ncm composite insertion torque.

When only 4 implants are used, the anterior-posterior spread becomes very important. In fact, the Skalac–Brunski model predicts that anterior-posterior spread is the most important factor in reducing implant stress.[24] Therefore, the surgeon should make an effort to gain as much anterior-posterior spread as possible, which favors angled implant placement. The factors then

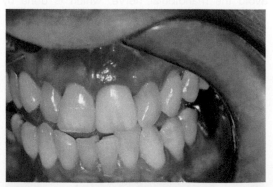

Fig. 16. A provisional restoration placed on the day of surgery.

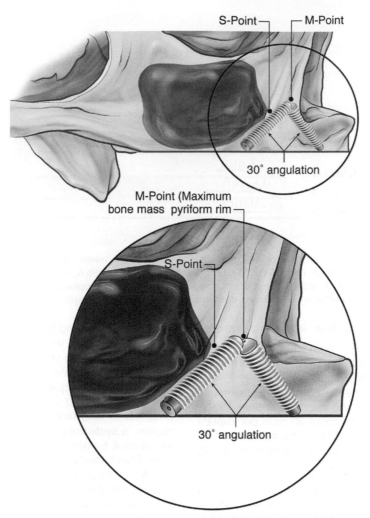

Fig. 18. A maxillary all-on-4 shelf shows sinus avoidance strategy using an M-shaped configuration with anchorage in maximum bone mass found between the sinus and nasal cavities.

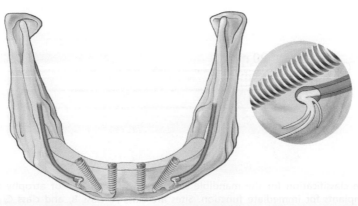

Fig. 19. A mandibular all-on-4 shelf benefits a nerve avoidance strategy as well as central placement of implants such that there is mature bone circumferentially around each implant.

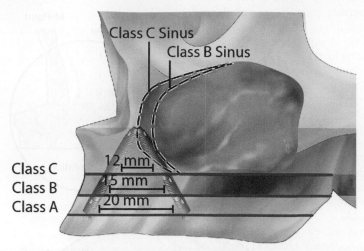

Fig. 20. All-on-4 site classification for the maxilla shows different levels of atrophy and therefore bone availability to fix implants for immediate function. Sites are class A, class B, and class C, depending on how much bone is available but also the position of the sinus. Interestingly, implants can be placed at almost the same position and angulation in all 3 classes with implants decreasing in length as bone deficiency progresses.

suggested for edentulous immediate function include the following:

1. Anterior posterior spread of 15 to 20 mm for maxilla and 12 to 20 mm for mandible
2. Cortical circumferential bone 4 mm per implant minimum maxilla and mandible
3. Insertion torque minimum 30 Ncm per implant or a composite of 120 Ncm for 4 implants
4. Implant number: Maxilla minimum of 4, mandible minimum of 3

These recommendations are guidelines, but when the surgeon is faced with the decision of what to do in certain situations, particularly after dental extraction and bone leveling is done, there must be systematic thinking to take advantage of available hard tissue structure to maximize potential for immediate function.

Whatever technique is used for immediate function, it should have a good chance to progress to long-term osseointegration. For this reason, a systematic approach is recommended for all-on-4 treatment that is based on available bone found *after* creation of the all-on-4 shelf to enable cortical fixation of implants even in settings of absence or near absence of bone. This site classification is illustrated in **Figs. 20** and **21**.

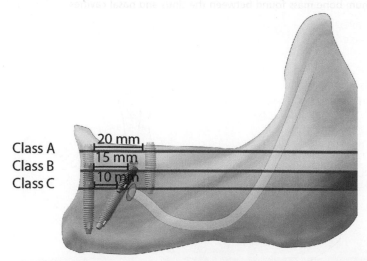

Fig. 21. All-on-4 site classification for the mandible showing different levels of atrophy and therefore bone availability to fix implants for immediate function. Sites are class A, class B, and class C, depending on how much bone is available but also the position of the mandibular nerve. Implants are placed in the same relative position anteriorly but vary posteriorly depending on bone availability above the nerve.

This illustration demonstrates a treatment-based classification according to the capacity for immediate functional loading of available bone.[25] The most common treatment sites are designated class A, B, and C. Class A sites have the most bone; class B has the next most bone, and class C has much less bone. Severe bone deficiency is seen in a fourth class, class D, which uses zygomatic fixtures for the maxilla; in the class D mandible, a requisite of only 3 fixtures. All of these approaches are based on the principles enumerated above, attempting to gain as much anterior-posterior spread as possible with adequate insertion torque for immediate function. Bone grafting is avoided except in the class C transsinus implant case.

Immediate functional loading whether for a single-tooth site or a complete arch requires a team approach, that is, both surgical and prosthetic expertise, which also means that the surgeon should know basic prosthetic principles to conceptualize treatment goals and intercept non-prosthetically sound efforts. The prosthodontist should be adept at surgical principles and help avoid treatment planning steps that lead to increased risk of surgical complications. When the team does not work well as a unit, the patient suffers the consequence and immediate function may fail. On the other hand, when surgical/prosthetic treatment is well-planned, well-coordinated, and well-executed, the interim and final results can be satisfying to all.

REFERENCES

1. Ferrus J, Cecchinato D, Pietursson EB, et al. Factors influencing ridge alterations following immediate implants placement into extraction sockets. Clin Oral Implants Res 2010;21(1):22–9.
2. Chen ST, Buser D. Esthetic outcomes following immediate and early implant placement in the anterior maxilla–a systematic review. Int J Oral Maxillofac Implants 2014;29(Suppl):186–215.
3. Cosyn J, Eghbali A, DeBruyn H, et al. Immediate single-tooth implants in the anterior maxilla: 3-year results of a case series on hard and soft tissue response and aesthetics. J Clin Periodontol 2011; 38(8):746–53.
4. Kassi B, Ivanovski S, Matheos N. Current perspectives on the role of ridge (socket) preservation procedures in dental implants treatment in the aesthetic zone. Aust Dent J 2014;59(1):48–56.
5. Vignoletti F, Sanz M. Immediate implants at fresh extraction sockets: from myth to reality. Periodontol 2000 2014;66(1):132–52.
6. Buser D, Chappuis V, Bornstein MM, et al. Long-term stability of contour augmentation with early implant placement following single tooth extraction in the esthetic zone: a prospective, cross-sectional study in 41 patients with a 5- to 9-year follow-up. J Periodontol 2013;84(11):1517–27.
7. Jempt T, Hager P. Early complete failures of fixed implant-supported prostheses in the edentulous maxilla: a three-year analysis of 17 consecutive cluster failure patients. Clin Implant Dent Relat Res 2006;8(2):77–86.
8. Hutton JE, Heath MR, Chai JY, et al. Factors related to success and failure rates at 3-year follow-up in a multicenter study of overdentures supported by Branemark implants. Int J Oral Maxillofac Implants 1995;10(1):33–42.
9. Schropp L, Wenzel A, Stavropoulos A. Early, delayed or late single implant placement: 10-year results from a randomized controlled clinical trial. Clin Oral Implants Res 2013;25(12):1359–65.
10. Morimoto T, Tsukiyama Y, Morimoto K, et al. Facial bone alterations on maxillary anterior single implants for immediate placement and provisionalization following extraction: a superimposed cone beam computed tomography study. Clin Oral Implants Res 2014;26(9). [Epub ahead of print].
11. Jensen OT, Adams MW, Cottam JR, et al. The all-on-4 shelf: maxilla. J Oral Maxillofac Surg 2010; 68(10):2520–7.
12. Al-Hezaimi K, Levi P, Rudy R, et al. An extraction socket classification developed using analysis of bone type and blood supply to the buccal bone in monkeys. Int J Periodontics Restorative Dent 2011; 31(4):421–7.
13. Cosyn J, Cleymaet R, De Bruyn H. Predictors of alveolar process remodeling following ridge preservation in high-risk patients. Clin Implant Dent Relat Res 2014;26(7). [Epub ahead of print].
14. Esposito M, Magharierth H, Grusovin MG, et al. Soft tissue management for dental implants: what are the most effective techniques? A Cochrane systematic review. Eur J Oral Implantol 2012;5(3):221–38.
15. Benic GI, Mir-Mari J, Hammerle CH. Loading protocols for single-implant crowns: a systematic review and meta-analysis. Int J Oral Maxillofac Implants 2014;29(Suppl):22–38.
16. Becker CM, Wilson TG Jr, Jensen OT. Minimum criteria for immediate provisionalization of single-tooth dental implants in extraction sites: a 1-year retrospective study of 100 consecutive cases. J Oral Maxillofac Surg 2011;69(2):491–7.
17. Malo P, Nobre Mde A, Lopes A. Immediate rehabilitation of completely edentulous arches with a four-implant prosthesis concept in difficult conditions: an open cohort study with a mean follow-up of 2 years. Int J Oral Maxillofac Implants 2012;27(5): 1177–90.
18. Jensen OT, Adams MW, Cottam JR, et al. The all-on-4 shelf: mandible. J Oral Maxillofac Surg 2011; 69(1):175–81.

19. Jensen OT, Adams MW. The maxillary M-4: a technical and biomechanical note for all-on-4 management of severe maxillary atrophy—report of 3 cases. J Oral Maxillofac Surg 2009;67(8):1739–44.

20. Jensen OT, Adams MW. Secondary stabilization of maxillary M-4 treatment with unstable implants for immediate function: biomechanical considerations and report of 10 cases after 1 year in function. Int J Oral Maxillofac Implants 2014;29(2): e232–40.

21. Jensen OT, Cottam J, Ringeman J. Avoidance of the mandibular nerve with implant placement: a new "mental loop". J Oral Maxillofac Surg 2011;69(6): 1540–3.

22. Trisi P, De Benedittis S, Perfectti G, et al. Primary stability, insertion torque and bone density of cylindrical implants and modem Branemark: is there a relationship? An in vitro study. Clin Oral Implants Res 2011; 22(5):567–70.

23. Liu C, Tsai MT, Huang HL, et al. Relation between insertion torque and bone implants contact percentage: an artificial bone study. Clin Oral Implants Res 2012;169(6):1679–84.

24. Jensen OT, Adams MW. Composite insertion torque for all-on-4 treatment, in press.

25. Jensen OT. Complete arch site classification for all-on-4 treatment. J Prosthet Dent 2014;112(4): 741–51.e2.

Esthetic Implant Site Development

Bach Le, DDS, MD, FICD, FACD*, Brady Nielsen, DDS

KEYWORDS

- Implant position • Implant angulation • Horizontal augmentation • Vertical augmentation
- Soft tissue augmentation • Emergence profile

KEY POINTS

- Bony support is critical for creating and maintaining esthetic and natural-appearing peri-implant soft tissue profiles.
- A variety of techniques have been shown to be effective for augmenting bone and soft tissue.
- Ideal implant position and angulation is critical for a natural-appearing outcome.
- Achieving an ideal esthetic result in the compromised site is often elusive and in many cases, impossible.

INTRODUCTION

The high predictability of implant-supported restorations has led to a shift in focus from success being solely equated with implant survival, yet most studies on implants fail to include criteria for esthetic success. It is reported that up to 16% of single-implant restorations in the esthetic zone fail for esthetic reasons,[1–3] with gingival recession and a lack of interdental papilla being the most common complications.[4] With proper treatment planning and execution, most complications can be avoided.

COMPREHENSIVE ESTHETIC EVALUATION

The pathway to esthetic success begins with an understanding of the features of an esthetic smile and an accurate diagnosis and treatment plan. The diagnostic process not only includes a thorough clinical and radiographic examination, but also an accurate determination of the patient's expectations.

Patient Expectations

The initial evaluation of the patient must include an understanding of the patient's expectations and a determination of whether these expectations can be met before treatment. Achieving an ideal esthetic result in the compromised site is often elusive and in many cases, impossible.[5] If the patient is found to have unrealistic expectations, a frank discussion is necessary to tailor their expectations to more realistic levels. An assessment of risk factors for implant failure and complications should be made. The potential for unexpected complications that can compromise the final result always exists with any surgical procedure and should be a part of the initial discussion on expectations.

It is also important to note that the esthetic outcomes perceived by the dental professionals and the patients do not always match.[6–9] Kokich and colleagues[9] compared the esthetic perception of dentists, orthodontist, and the layperson on various parameters. They did this by altering

Disclosure Statement: The authors are not employed or compensated in any form by any implant company and do not endorse a specific product brand.
Department of Oral & Maxillofacial Surgery, The Herman Ostrow School of Dentistry of USC, Los Angeles County/USC Medical Center, 1983 Marengo St, Los Angeles, CA 90033, USA
* Corresponding author.
E-mail address: leb97201@yahoo.com

Oral Maxillofacial Surg Clin N Am 27 (2015) 283–311
http://dx.doi.org/10.1016/j.coms.2015.01.009

various parameters and asking each group to judge the esthetic perception of these altered parameters (eg, teeth length, gingival margin level, papilla height). According to Kokich and colleagues,[9] patients consider a discrepancy in gingival margin of more than 2 mm to be unesthetic, similar to those of general dentists. Conversely, the investigators found that although dentists had very low tolerance for any discrepancy in papilla height, most laypersons were not able to differentiate a severely compromised papilla height. Tymstra and colleagues[5] reported the results of placing 2 adjacent maxillary implants after autogenous block grafts in 10 consecutive patients. The investigators reported that in 40% of their cases, there was an absence of the interdental papilla. Interestingly, all the patients in this study reported that their results were "acceptable" or better, supporting the findings of the study by Kokich and colleagues.[9]

The Esthetic Smile

A variety of parameters exist when defining the esthetic smile. These requirements exist for both the static and dynamic states.[10] Some of the general guidelines include the following:

- Maxillary incisor show at rest of 2 to 4 mm[10]
- Full animation displays 75% to 100% of maxillary incisors with 1 to 2 mm of gingival display[10,11]
- Maxillary anterior teeth follow the Golden Proportion: when viewed from the facial aspect, the width of each subsequent tooth should be 60% of the adjacent, mesial tooth[12]
- The Recurring Esthetic Dental Proportion: when viewed from the facial aspect, the successive width proportion should remain constant while moving away from the midline[13,14]
- Maxillary central incisors should have a length of 10 to 11 mm and their width should be 75% to 80% of the length
- Maxillary central incisor widths should be 2 to 3 mm greater than the lateral incisor and 1.0 to 1.5 mm greater than the canine
- Maxillary central incisors and canines are longer than the lateral incisor by 1.0 to 1.5 mm
- The gingival zenith of central incisors and canines should coincide, and that of the lateral incisors should be located 0.5 to 1.0 mm more coronal[11]
- The outline of maxillary anterior teeth incisal edges should mirror the lower lip line
- The gingival margin of the maxillary anterior teeth runs parallel with the upper lip line[11]
- Adequate quality and quantity of keratinized soft tissue must be present[11]

- Natural sulcular and papilla forms around teeth are present with no black triangles[15,16]
- The vermilion border is most highly defined centrally near the philtrum and is supported by the dentoalveolar anatomy of the anterior maxilla[11]

During treatment planning, each of the parameters contributing to an esthetic smile should be considered when the restorative dentist fabricates a diagnostic wax-up with teeth in ideal positions. The starting point for determining tooth position is the maxillary central incisor edge position. Once incisor edge position is determined, it is possible to determine the desired gingival levels based on appropriate teeth length. In evaluating the compromised edentulous or partially edentulous segment, an existing removable partial denture or a clear radiographic and/or surgical guide may be used to determine the ideal maxillary incisal edge position (**Fig. 1**).

Establishing the appropriate gingival level during the diagnostic examination will determine if any hard or soft tissue augmentation or reduction will be required to achieve ideal teeth length and proportion in the final restoration.

Radiographic Examination

Cone-beam computed tomography (CBCT) has become an integral part in 3-dimensional dental implant treatment planning. It allows evaluation of bone quality, alveolar ridge topography, soft tissue thickness, proximity to vital anatomic structures, and fabrication of surgical guides. CBCT is preferably done with the patient wearing a surgical guide with radiopaque markers to indicate the ideal position and angulation of the planned implant fixtures and restorations. The imaging will reveal the relationship between the existing alveolar housing and the ideal position of the final restoration. This will help determine whether or not hard tissue augmentation is required, and in which dimension. **Table 1** provides a summary of techniques for evaluating ideal tooth position in relation to existing bone and soft tissue level.

Clinical Examination

A comprehensive clinical examination is primarily aimed at determining the hard and soft tissue status at the planned implant site. The examination should consist of an assessment of the soft tissues and alveolar width and height in the facial-lingual and vertical dimensions. The soft tissue evaluation includes measurements of soft tissue thickness, papilla height, gingival margin level, and width of the keratinized tissue band. Evaluate for collapse of the facial plate or tissue loss in the vertical

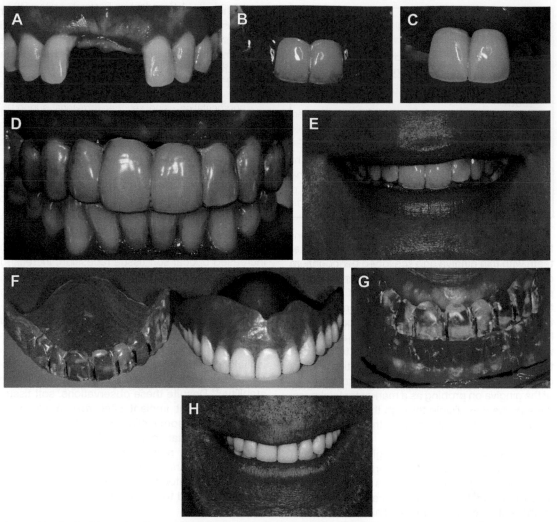

Fig. 1. (*A–H*) Ideal incisal edge position and evaluation of edentulous segment. An Essix appliance, existing removable prosthesis, or a clear radiographic and/or surgical guide may be used to evaluate the need to augment the edentulous alveolar segment and to determine the ideal incisal edge position. (*A*) Edentulous segment. (*B*) Essix appliance. (*C*) Removable appliance. (*D*) Essix appliance used to evaluate the need for alveolar augmentation. (*E*) Essix appliance used to determine ideal incisal edge position. (*F*) Surgical guide and removable prosthesis. (*G*) Clear surgical guide. (*H*) Existing removable. (*Courtesy of* Bach Le, DDS, MD, Los Angeles, CA.)

Table 1 Techniques for evaluating ideal tooth position in relation to existing bone and soft tissue level	
Existing removable prosthesis or Surgical Guide Try-In	Quickly determines ideal tooth position in relation to existing hard and soft tissues
Computed tomography imaging with surgical guide and radiopaque markers	Reveals quantity of existing hard tissue and relationship to ideal tooth position

dimension. When possible, compare the planned edentulous implant site to the existing contralateral tooth or teeth segments in the anterior esthetic zone. Comparing gingival margin levels, papilla forms, and presence of keratinized tissue will quickly make the implant surgeon aware of any discrepancies and deficiencies. The use of photographic records in the initial workup can serve as a valuable tool for proper treatment planning in the esthetic zone.

Gingival biotype
Patients exhibit differences in their gingival phenotypes, often termed "gingival biotypes" (**Table 2**).[17]

Table 2 Gingival biotypes	
Biotype I: Thin Gingival Biotype	**Biotype II: Thick Gingival Biotype**
Triangular-shaped tooth	Square-shaped tooth
Scalloped and thin periodontium	Flat and thick periodontium
Interproximal contact area in the coronal 1/3 of the crown	Interproximal contact area in the middle 1/3 of the crown
Long and thin papilla	Short and wide papilla

Most patients will fall into 2 categories: slender teeth with thin gingiva and scalloped periodontium or square teeth with thick gingiva and blunted periodontium (**Fig. 2**).[17,18] In a study of 100 volunteers, De Rouck and colleagues[18–21] demonstrated that approximately one-third of the patients exhibited thin biotype, which was usually associated with female patients. Two-thirds were thicker biotypes usually associated with male patients. They classified the 2 biotypes by using the translucency of the gingiva on probing as a marker for thickness; if the probe was visible through the facial gingival tissue, this was considered a thin biotype, and conversely.[18]

Much consideration has been given to the thickness of the gingiva and its importance in implant dentistry. The thinner biotype is more prone to recession and loss of interdental papilla.[18,22–24] In the esthetic zone, some clinicians advocate the routine use of connective tissue grafts to transform thin biotypes into thicker tissue for enhanced esthetic outcomes.[25,26] Studies have shown that the thickness of bone around implants can affect the overlying soft tissue profile. Le and Borzabadi-Farahani[27] showed a high correlation between labial crestal soft tissue thickness and underlying bone thickness, demonstrating that soft tissue thickness can be heavily influenced by the labial bone thickness (**Fig. 3**).

In other words, the thicker the bone, the thicker the crestal labial soft tissue around implants and vice versa. Based on these findings, soft tissue augmentation may not be necessary if adequate labial crestal bone thickness exists (>2 mm). If an implant site exhibits a thin biotype, a connective tissue graft or bone augmentation should be considered either before or at the time of implant placement.

The keratinized band
Different opinions exist as to whether a lack of keratinized tissue may jeopardize the maintenance of the soft tissue health around dental implants.[28–30] Some investigators have reported that implants with a reduced width of less than 2 mm of peri-implant keratinized mucosa are associated with increased buccal soft tissue recession, increased alveolar bone loss, more plaque accumulation, increased bleeding, and poorer soft tissue health.[31,32] Others have not found similar correlations. Two recent literature reviews concluded that the lack of keratinized tissue around implants does not influence implant survival[33] and evidence is lacking to support the need for keratinized tissues around implants to maintain health and tissue stability.[34] Despite these observations, soft tissue augmentation at implant sites may need to be considered in some clinical situations in which adequate crestal bone thickness cannot be achieved. Other reasons for an adequate keratinized tissue band include the need to improve the esthetic outcome,[35] to facilitate restorative procedures, and to help maintain oral hygiene.

The interdental papilla
The development of papilla adjacent to the implant is an integral part of dental implant therapy. This will result in a more natural, youthful-looking dental restoration, which is critical in the esthetic zone. Predictable papilla formation is dependent on the gingival biotype and bony attachment of the adjacent teeth rather than the tooth to be extracted.[25,36] Thick gingival tissue can tolerate more bone loss on the adjacent tooth and still maintain papilla

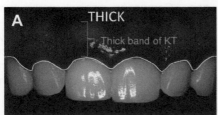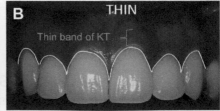

Fig. 2. Gingival biotype. Most patients will fall into 2 categories: slender teeth with thin gingiva and scalloped periodontium or square teeth with thick gingiva and blunted periodontium. (*A*) Thick gingival biotype. (*B*) Thin gingival biotype. (*Courtesy of* Bach Le, DDS, MD, Los Angeles, CA.)

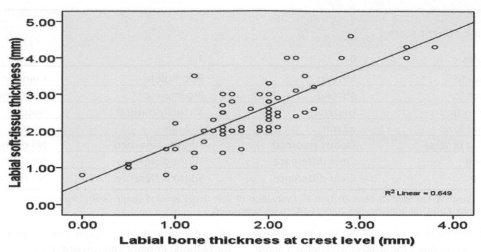

Fig. 3. Labial soft tissue thickness and labial bone thickness. Linear correlation between labial crestal soft tissue thickness and underlying bone thickness. (*Courtesy of* Bach Le, DDS, MD, Los Angeles, CA.)

compared with thinner biotypes.[24,37] Single-tooth defects often have more predictable papilla form than multiple-teeth defects, because the presence of adjacent natural teeth allows for retention of the interproximal height of bone. When adjacent teeth are lost, the osseous scallop is lost, causing a reduction in interproximal papilla height.[38,39]

Furhauser and colleagues[40] described a method for objectively measuring 7 parameters for gingival esthetics around a restored single-tooth implant crown called the pink esthetic score. Each variable was graded with a score of 0 to 2 for each variable (**Fig. 4**, **Table 3**). They found that the papilla was the variable to most often receive a score of 2, suggesting that for a single-unit implant restoration, it is not a difficult esthetic variable to achieve.

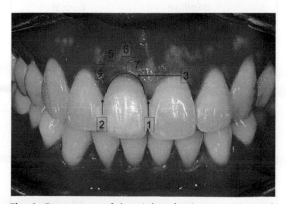

Fig. 4. Parameters of the pink esthetic score. The pink esthetic score provides a reproducible method for evaluating papilla form as well as other soft tissue variables listed in **Table 3**. (*Courtesy of* Bach Le, DDS, MD, Los Angeles, CA.)

The presence of intercrestal bone is a predictable indicator of whether papilla regeneration is plausible.[37,41–43] The distance between the contact point between the crowns and the interproximal bone crest influences the papilla fill. One study reported that when this distance was 5 mm or less, complete papilla fill was always found, whereas unpredictable papilla formation was seen in sites when the distance was greater than 5 mm.[42] Because it is difficult to predictably graft bone or soft tissue to gain adequate papilla height, this limitation should be anticipated so that patient expectations can be appropriately addressed. Considerations should be given to broadening the proximal contact point of the affected teeth to prevent the dreaded "black triangle" or extraction of the compromised tooth followed by bone augmentation.

Gingival level

Because gingival recession is possible after implant placement,[44–46] it is critical to assess the gingival margin height of the tooth or implant site. This margin is usually dictated by the underlying facial bone level. A free gingival margin that lies coronal to the planned restorative margin offers some insurance against recession and is considered more favorable. In clinical cases in which the gingival margin is in an unfavorable position, techniques such as guided bone regeneration (GBR) with coronal tissue advancement to bring the gingival margin and bone into a more coronal level before implant placement should be considered.[47,48]

In contrast to the higher scores for papilla height at single-unit implant restorations, Furhauser and colleagues[40] noted consistently lower scores for

Table 3
The pink esthetic score

Variables	0	1	2
Papilla - M	Missing	Incomplete	Complete
Papilla - D	Missing	Incomplete	Complete
Tissue contours	Unnatural	Virtually natural	Natural
Gingival level	>2 mm	1–2 mm	<1 mm
Alveolar process	Clearly resorbed	Slightly resorbed	No difference
Coloring	Clear difference	Slight difference	No difference
Texture	Clear difference	Slight difference	No difference

From Furhauser R, Florescu D, Benesch T, et al. Evaluation of soft tissue around single-tooth implant crowns: the pink esthetic score. Clin Oral Implants Res 2005;16:642; with permission.

gingival margin level and soft tissue color. These were the parameters most likely to receive a score of 0. Only 44% of single-unit implant restorations displayed a gingival margin level within 1 mm of the contralateral reference tooth. The poor esthetic outcome may be due to a variety of factors, including crestal bone remodeling to establish a biological width,[49] soft tissue recession, and a thin facial plate prone to resorption.

Palacci and Ericsson Alveolar Ridge Classification System

Many classification systems exist for assessing the hard and soft tissue defects.[50,51] Palacci and Ericsson described an alveolar ridge classification system for the anterior maxilla according to vertical and horizontal loss in both hard and soft tissue (**Table 4**).[11]

The benefit of such a classification system is that it provides prognostic and treatment guidelines. The Palacci and Ericsson system includes the following key points:

- A single surgical procedure can improve the classification by only 1 level
- A series of surgical procedures are required to improve by multiple classification levels
- A total of 5 to 6 mm of apparent tissue height can be gained through a series of surgical steps
  - 4 to 5 mm of total tissue height can be obtained through bone and soft tissue augmentation
    - 2 to 3 mm of bone height can be obtained
    - 2 mm of soft tissue height can be obtained
  - Crown lengthening may provide an additional 1 to 2 mm of height

The principles conveyed by the Palacci and Ericsson classification system can be simplified by the following general guidelines that apply to all patients requiring augmentation procedures for esthetic implant site development:

- When the bony structure is inadequate, multiple hard and soft tissue augmentation procedures are often required
- When the bony structure is adequate, soft tissue augmentation still may be indicated to achieve the ideal esthetic result
- Esthetic implant site development requires a significantly greater time commitment and number of augmentation procedures for sites with multiple missing teeth compared with a site with a single missing tooth

Table 4
Palacci and Ericsson alveolar ridge classification system

Vertical Loss		Horizontal Loss	
Class I	Intact or slightly reduced papillae	Class A	Intact or slightly reduced buccal tissues
Class II	Limited loss of papillae (<50%)	Class B	Limited loss of buccal tissues
Class III	Severe loss of papillae	Class C	Severe loss of buccal tissues
Class IV	Absence of papillae (edentulous ridge)	Class D	Extreme loss of buccal tissue, often combined with limited amount of attached mucosa

From Palacci P, Nowzari H. Soft tissue enhancement around dental implants. Periodontol 2000;47:113–32; with permission.

TREATMENT PLANNING

The greatest determinants of the esthetic result are surgical in nature, including the techniques used for hard and soft tissue augmentation procedures, implant placement, and implant uncovering.[52] Often times a patient will present with a combination of hard and soft tissue deficits. These cases require a staged surgical approach aimed at addressing the bony defects before beginning any soft tissue intervention. Many cases will even need some procedures performed multiple times to achieve the best result.

Preservation of Hard and Soft Tissues

Preservation of the existing tissues should be the primary goal of any treatment plan. The best way to obtain adequate hard and soft tissues for an esthetic implant site is to prevent its loss following tooth extraction. Early preservation and augmentation is important, as approximately 3 to 4 mm of bone loss occurs in the first 6 months after extraction of a tooth.[53–58] Socket grafting for ridge preservation has been advocated to decrease the amount of bone loss after tooth extraction.[59–62] Comparative research has shown that patients who underwent a ridge preservation procedure sustained significantly less resorption than patients who were not treated.[55,59,62,63] Ridge preservation will help facilitate prosthetically driven implant placement. It also may obviate the need to undergo more invasive bone augmentation procedures and thereby shorten treatment duration.

Implants placed into extraction sockets have been advocated to maintain the alveolar bone volume after extraction. Although immediate implants have been shown to integrate with high success rates similar to implants placed with a delayed approach,[24,25,44,64–67] studies have shown that implants placed into extraction sockets do not necessarily prevent alveolar ridge changes,[65–67] and may often be subject to some labial gingival recession (**Fig. 5**).[24,44–46,68] In a retrospective analysis of 42 single-tooth implants placed in the esthetic zone, a significant change in crown height due to marginal tissue recession of approximately 1 mm was noted.[68] Thin tissue biotypes showed slightly greater recession than thick-tissue biotypes.

Conversely, in a randomized control study, Block and colleagues[36] found no statistically significant differences in crestal or interproximal bone levels when comparing immediate or delayed implant placement with immediate provisionalization in the anterior maxilla. The investigators concluded that immediate implant placement with provisionalization resulted in approximately

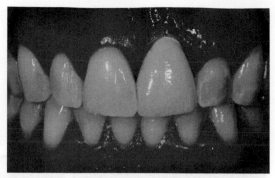

Fig. 5. Labial gingival recession. Labial gingival recession 1 year after implant placement. (*Courtesy of* Bach Le, DDS, MD, Los Angeles, CA.)

1 mm less facial gingival recession compared with that in the delayed group. The investigators also noted that papilla formation was dependent on the attachment of the adjacent teeth, and elevating the papilla off the alveolar ridge did not affect subsequent papilla formation. Because it was not evaluated in this study, it is unclear how biotype delineation may have affected the results.

When multiple teeth are indicated for extraction, a staged approach using strategic extractions of selected teeth and fabrication of either a tooth-borne or implant-borne temporary fixed partial denture will help to decrease bone loss and maintain the supporting bone and tissue architecture (**Fig. 6**).[11,69] In a controlled animal study, Favero and colleagues[70] demonstrated that tooth extraction next to a socket into which an immediate implant is placed caused more bone loss in both buccolingual and mesiodistal dimensions compared with sites adjacent to a maintained tooth.

Defect Configuration

One of the primary goals of esthetic implant site development[71] is the successful placement and long-term maintenance of bone graft material in labial crestal contour of the peri-implant region. This region is largely responsible for the labial soft tissue contour and long-term stability of the gingival margin level. With bone augmentation, graft migration and resorption from this area often result in unesthetic tissue recession. The challenge in maintaining this bone depends on a number of critical factors related to defect configuration.

Width of edentulous span

Single-tooth defects have a much better esthetic prognosis than multiple-teeth defects.[72] This concept is also true for bone augmentation. Particulate grafts in wider edentulous spans are more prone to migration due to wide flap elevation.

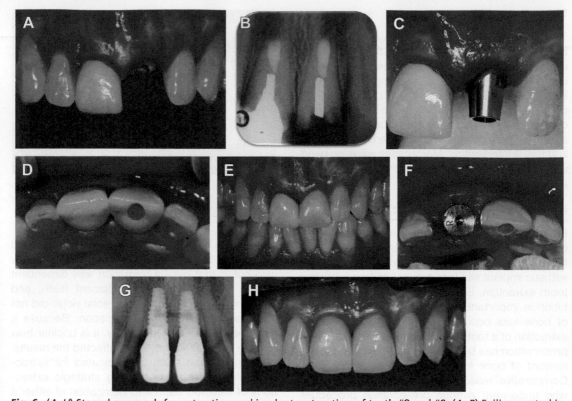

Fig. 6. (*A–H*) Staged approach for extraction and implant restoration of teeth #8 and #9. (*A, B*) Failing central incisors before implant restoration. (*C–E*) Extraction of the left central incisor with immediate implant placement and provisional restoration. (*C*) Staged implant. (*D, E*) Temporary restoration. (*F*) Staged implant. Four months later, extraction of the right central incisor was performed with immediate implant placement and provisional restoration. (*G, H*) Final restoration at 3-year follow-up with radiograph showing preserved gingival architecture. (*H*) Preservation of soft tissue architecture using staged approach. (*Courtesy of* Bach Le, DDS, MD, Los Angeles, CA.)

Wider defects often require the use of containment barrier or space maintenance, such as a mesh or a membrane with tacks to contain the bone graft material (**Fig. 7**).

Number of walls

New bone formation mainly depends on the surface area of exposed bone and bone marrow because the osteogenic and angiogenic cells

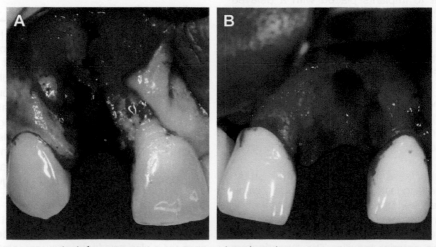

Fig. 7. Narrow versus wide defects. Particulate grafts in wider edentulous spans are more prone to migration due to wide flap elevation. Wider defects often require the use of containment barrier to contain the bone graft material. (*A*) Narrow buccal wall defect. (*B*) Wide buccal wall defect. (*Courtesy of* Bach Le, DDS, MD, Los Angeles, CA.)

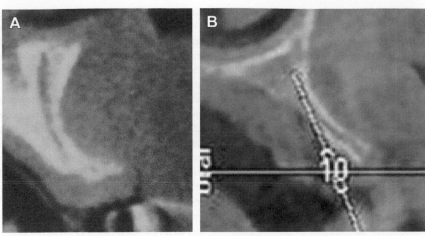

Fig. 8. Defect with walls and defect without walls. (*A*) Favorable defect. Horizontal defect with bony concavities to contain graft material. (*B*) Unfavorable defect. Horizontal defect with 1 wall and no bony concavities are much more challenging to graft with particulate graft material due to apical migration. (*Courtesy of* Bach Le, DDS, MD, Los Angeles, CA.)

that form new bone reside in the bone marrow.[73] The healing potential of a given defect increases with each bony wall available.[74] The number of bony walls available in a defect has a significant influence on the success of the bone augmentation procedure. Three to 4 wall defects have a better prognosis for containment of graft material within the skeletal borders with minimal migration and space maintenance. Defects with fewer walls are more difficult and often require additional graft procedures to attain the optimal result.

Type of defect

Horizontal defects with bony concavities to contain graft material have better prognosis than those with no walls (**Fig. 8**). Defects with vertical components are the most difficult due to the difficulty in space maintenance. The use of space maintenance devices, such as titanium mesh[75,76] or tenting screws,[77] is recommended in these defects. Distraction osteogenesis and segmental osteotomies also have been described for the management of these defects.[78,79]

Management of Horizontal Defects

Most postextraction losses of alveolar ridge dimensions occur in the horizontal (width) rather than the vertical (height) plane.[53] Even when there is adequate bone to place implants, irregular ridge anatomy that is not corrected can result in an unnatural appearance of the final restoration (**Fig. 9**). Bone augmentation before or simultaneously with implant placement may allow for better implant position. Additionally, the augmented bone will correct ridge contour defects for a

more natural-looking restoration and increase facial bone support for long-term peri-implant soft tissue stability.[80,81]

Single-tooth replacement in sites with horizontal defects must follow the same initial guiding principles discussed previously. Important considerations are the level of the gingival margin (as this is dictated by the facial bone level), bone attachment of the adjacent teeth (as this will dictate the presence or absence of final papillary height), and thickness of the tissue biotype.

Many techniques have been described for lateral ridge augmentation. These include GBR, ridge expansion/splitting, autogenous onlay block grafting, and connective tissue grafting.[82–91]

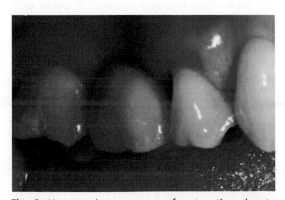

Fig. 9. Unnatural appearance of restoration due to collapsed buccal alveolus. Even when there is adequate bone to place implants, irregular ridge anatomy that is not corrected can result in an unnatural appearance of the final restoration. (*Courtesy of* Bach Le, DDS, MD, Los Angeles, CA.)

Particulate grafting with guided bone regeneration

Particulated bone has been used for horizontal augmentation with good success for mild-to-moderately sized defects.[91,92] Using the soft tissue matrix theory, meshes, reinforced membranes, screws, dental implants, cortical bone, and the graft itself have been used to maintain this expanded pocket.[71,77,93–95] A tenting mechanism to prevent collapse of the soft tissue can be extremely advantageous when augmenting vertical or large horizontal defects.

Block and Degen[86] described a minimally invasive tunneling technique using mineralized particulate allograft to horizontally augment partially edentulous defects for successful implant placement. However, a disadvantage of the tunneling technique is that it can be difficult to position and maintain the graft in a coronal position to augment the peri-implant soft tissue. Additional bone grafting is usually necessary at the time of implant placement to address this issue.[71] Maintaining the graft in the crestal area is important in long-term peri-implant soft tissue stability.[80,96]

Ridge augmentation exclusively using particulate grafts is extremely technique-sensitive and operator-dependent. Predictability of lateral ridge augmentation using particulate grafts is largely dependent on the ability to stabilize and maintain the soft tissue matrix. Maintenance of this space becomes more difficult with long edentulous spans or when there is inadequate basal bone support. The analogy of building a sandcastle applies with the use of particulate grafts for ridge augmentation. When building a sandcastle, a wide base is needed first to support the sand at the highest portion (**Fig. 10**). Without adequate basal bone support, the most coronal portion of the graft often migrates apically. If using only particulate graft for larger width correction, basal bone width can be augmented first using a tunneling approach[86] or an open approach. The remaining defect can be further augmented at the time of implant placement.[71,97,98]

"Esthetic contour graft": single-stage implants with simultaneous guided bone regeneration

GBR has been proven experimentally and clinically to promote osseous regeneration and to preserve a large percentage of grafted material.[99–102] The traditional GBR procedure is performed as a staged approach with a second surgical procedure to place the implant. If simultaneous bone grafting is performed, it is usually done with the implant submerged underneath the soft tissue. Le and Burstein[71] described a simultaneous bone grafting with implant placement in a nonsubmerged single-stage protocol using a healing abutment. This approach offers many advantages. The single-stage protocol minimizes compression and migration of particulate graft material and it allows the bony and soft tissue architecture to develop around the healing abutment during the healing phase. A large-diameter healing abutment, in a single-stage placement protocol, provides tenting of the peri-implant soft tissue and results in less apical migration of graft material. This improves the prognosis by safeguarding the width and height of the remaining crestal bone. Grafting at the time of implant placement also takes advantage of the regional acceleratory phenomenon[103] that is induced by the trauma of implant placement, leading to a reduced healing time.

Simultaneous bone grafting with 2-stage implant placement has shown promising results.[104] Le and Borzabadi-Farahani[105] assessed the outcome of single-stage (nonsubmerged) implant placement and simultaneous augmentation of 156 sites with vertical buccal defect using a mineralized particulate allograft covered with a collagen membrane. The vertical buccal defects were classified as small (<3 mm in depth), medium (3–5 mm in depth), and large (>5 mm in depth). The initial vertical buccal wall defect was recorded by measuring the amount of vertical implant platform's rough surface exposure after implants were placed. Sectional CBCT scans were used at 36 months after graft healing. The site of the original vertical bone defect was evaluated for the presence of any residual vertical bone defect. The results showed the presence of bone in 100.0% and 79.3% of small and medium-sized vertical defects, respectively. Large-size defects showed only partial improvement without any complete correction. Single-stage implant placement with simultaneous bone grafting to support the soft tissue margin showed promising outcomes in correcting vertical buccal wall defects smaller than 3 mm (**Fig. 11**).[105]

Another recently published article by Jensen and colleagues[106] analyzed the long-term stability of contour augmentation during early implant placement (implant placement after 6–8 weeks of healing following tooth extraction) based on human biopsies harvested from the esthetic zone. The implant placement was performed with simultaneous contour augmentation using deproteinized bovine bone mineral (DBBM) and a collagen barrier membrane. The biopsies were subjected to histologic and histomorphometric analysis. Results showed that the biopsies consisted of 32.0% ± 9.6% DBBM particles and 40.6% ± 14.6% mature bone; 70.3% ± 14.5% of the DBBM particle surfaces were covered with bone. They concluded that osseointegrated

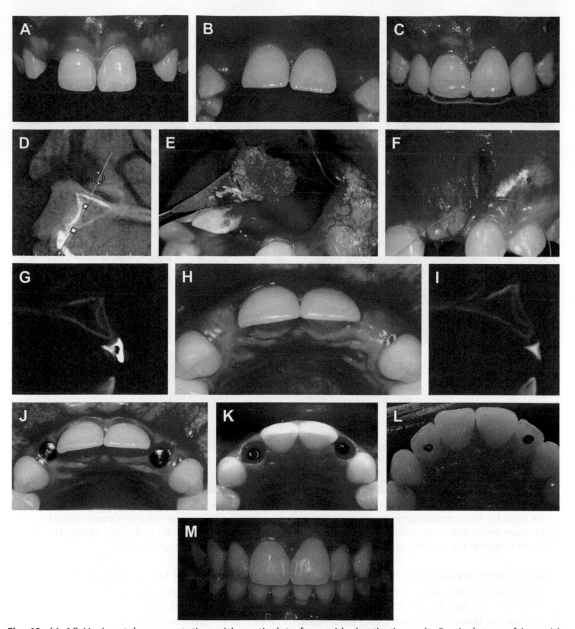

Fig. 10. (*A–M*) Horizontal augmentation with particulate for an ideal esthetic result. Particulate grafting with GBR principles can be used for horizontal augmentation so long as an adequate bony foundation is already present to support the particulate graft. (*A, B*) Alveolar width defect. (*C*) Radiopaque Essix appliance. (*D*) Radiographic marker. (*E*) Particulate graft placement. (*F*) Closure over membrane. (*G*) Site augmentation of #7. (*H*) Clinically evident augmentation. (*I*) Site augmentation of #10. (*J*) Implant position. (*K*) Soft tissue thickness. (*L, M*) Final restoration. (*Courtesy of* Bach Le, DDS, MD, Los Angeles, CA.)

DBBM particles do not tend to undergo substitution over time, confirming previous findings. This low substitution rate supports the clinically and radiographically documented long-term stability of contour augmentation using a combination of autogenous bone chips, DBBM particles, and a collagen membrane.[107]

The success of the "esthetic contour graft" concept is dependent on multiple important variables. These include defect configuration, flap design, space maintenance, graft selection, membrane selection, and implant position. Each of these principles plays a critical role and can influence the success or failure of the procedure.

Flap design

Minimizing flap exposure to maximize vascular supply to the surgical site while creating adequate

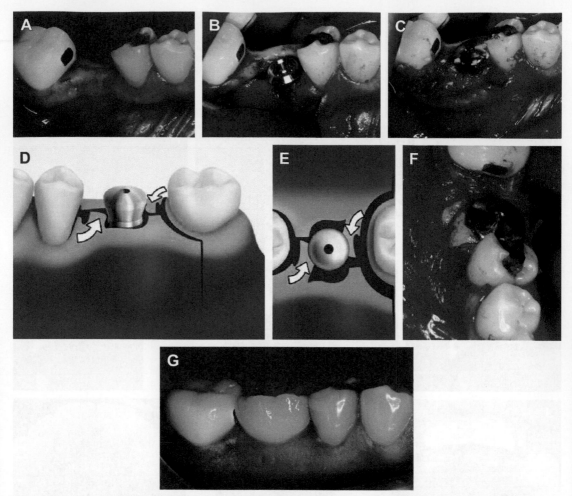

Fig. 11. Simultaneous implant placement and horizontal augmentation. Particulate grafting with GBR principles can be used for horizontal augmentation with simultaneous implant placement to correct small vertical defects. (*A*) Alveolar width defect. (*B*) Implant placement. (*C*) Horizontal augmentation. (*D, E*) Incision design. (*F*) Closure. (*G*) Natural-appearing final restoration. (*Courtesy of* Bach Le, DDS, MD, Los Angeles, CA.)

access for graft placement can be delicate. Surgical exposure can be limited to a flapless approach when there is no anticipation for bone augmentation (adequate bone width, height, and keratinized tissue width). A flapless protocol offers many advantages, including faster recovery, less postoperative discomfort, decreased crestal bone loss, and decreased tissue recession. With increasing defect size, surgical exposure will require an incision design using a sulcular flap, envelope flap with extension to adjacent teeth, or vertical releasing incisions. For small ridge defects (<2 mm), a flapless or sulcular incision may be adequate. For larger defects, an open-book flap design may be used to enhance visualization and access to the graft site (**Fig. 12**). It is important to achieve tension-free adaptation of wound margins during wound closure. Raising a flap for correction of the anatomic defect requires incising or scoring

the periosteum for tension-free expansion of the soft tissue matrix. In addition to allowing primary tension-free wound closure, scoring of the periosteum also promotes angiogenesis by creating bleeding into the graft.[108]

Open-book flap procedure

Grafting of labial wall defects using GBR has been described to correct postextraction defects using either a flapless approach, which involves positioning a barrier membrane within the socket and packing mineralized allograft into the socket,[109] or with flap elevation. Although a flapless surgery can be easier to perform, bone regeneration will be limited to the confines of the socket, and will likely be subjected to resorption past the confines of the labial wall during the natural resorption and remodeling processes.[64] As a result, anatomic contours may not be achieved and future bone

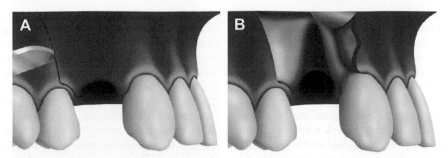

Fig. 12. Open-book flap design. The open-book flap design should be used for large defects to improve visualization and access to the graft site. (*A*) Incision design. (*B*) Open-book flap elevation. (*Courtesy of* Bach Le, DDS, MD, Los Angeles, CA.)

grafting still may be needed. When labial wall defects are present, grafting with an open-flap approach is recommended and will yield predictable peri-implant tissue and bone stability.[71,97,110]

The open-book flap is developed with a crestal incision made slightly lingual to the ridge midline to preserve an adequate amount of keratinized tissue in the flap (**Fig. 13**). This is followed by a distal, curvilinear, vertical incision that follows the gingival margin of the distal tooth. A wide subperiosteal reflection is made to expose 2 to 3 times the treatment area, and then the papilla is reflected on the mesial side of the edentulous site. During implant placement, the implant's restorative platform is positioned to the desired level, and a healing cap is attached to the implant. The peri-implant

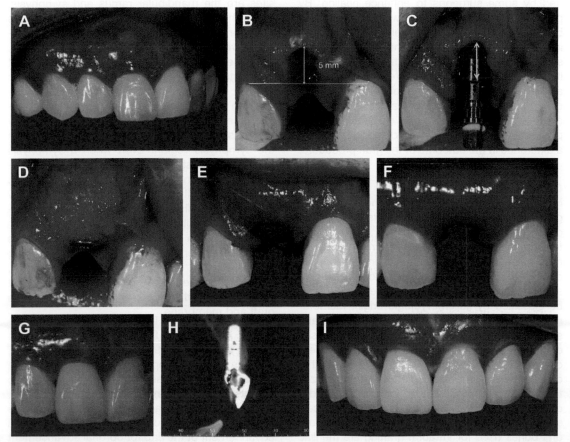

Fig. 13. (*A–I*) Open-book flap design and surgical technique. Open-book flap design with esthetic contour graft and nonsubmerged closure around healing abutment. (*A*) Preoperative. (*B*) Open-book flap. (*C*) Implant depth. (*D*) Contour graft. (*E*) Nonsubmerged. (*F*) Three months postoperative. (*G*) Provisional. (*H*) Five-year radiograph. (*I*) Five years postoperative. (*Courtesy of* Bach Le, DDS, MD, Los Angeles, CA.)

soft tissue is released and advanced by scoring the periosteum so that a tension-free closure is achieved around the neck of the implant. This is done because moderate graft resorption will occur if there is inadequate tissue seal around the implant neck or if tension-free closure is not achieved. To induce bleeding in the graft site, perform a periosteum release as the last step just before graft placement. Pack human mineralized bone allograft into the defect and overcontour by approximately 20% to 30% to compensate for anticipated apical migration and resorption of the material. Before surgery, hydrate the allograft according to the manufacturer's directions and mix with the patient's blood, which serves as a coagulant. After grafting, cover the allograft with a resorbable membrane, and attach a wide healing abutment to the implant. Finally, approximate the soft tissues and suture around the healing abutment. This creates a tenting effect over the allograft and, together with the healing abutment, helps to hold the particulate material in place.

Perforating the recipient bone bed is recommended by some surgeons to enhance healing. By perforating the cortical bone with a small round bur, the marrow cavity is opened and bleeding into the defect is induced. Animal studies have shown that perforations in cortical bone improve healing in a membrane-protected defect.[111,112] It also was shown that larger perforations were associated with prompter bone formation.[103] The senior author (Bach Le) of this article does not routinely perforate the recipient bone bed and has not seen a difference in the outcome of the graft procedure.

Onlay grafting

Many clinicians have reported on the use of autogenous bone,[83,94,113–120] allografts,[86,121] xenografts,[104,122,123] and alloplastic[124,125] onlay grafts to augment the width of the atrophic ridge for placement and successful integration of endosseous implants. Autogenous bone, considered to be the gold standard for grafting hard tissue defects,[126,127] can be classified by its embryologic origin. Membranous bones, including the calvarium, ramus, and symphysis, are formed by intramembranous ossification. This process involves embryonic mesenchymal cells differentiating into osteoblasts that can synthesize an osteoid matrix that mineralizes to form hard bone. Bone also is formed by endochondral ossification of cartilage at the epiphyseal surface of long bones. Two examples of endochondral bones used for intraoral grafting are the iliac crest and tibial plateau.

In reviewing the literature on graft survival,[128,129] membranous bone grafts retained greater than 80% of their original volume and had been replaced by new bone, whereas iliac (endochondral) bone had undergone 65% to 88% resorption. In addition to the higher resorption rate of iliac crest grafts, other disadvantages include the high costs of hospitalization, risks of general anesthesia, and morbidity of the procedure.[116,119,130] Conversely, mandibular symphysis and ramus bone appear to undergo less resorption because of the thick cortical layer and their rigid structure.[116,119,131] Other advantages of intraoral donor sites include conventional access for surgeons familiar with intraoral anatomy, less anesthetic risk, reduced operative time due to close proximity of donor and recipient sites, and no cutaneous scars.[131–133] It can also be ideally done as an outpatient surgery, thereby decreasing the overall costs of the procedure.

Various intraoral sites have been described for graft donor sites. These include the mandibular ramus,[83,114,115,134] symphysis,[135,136] maxillary tuberosity,[75,137] maxillary and mandibular tori,[138] and osteotomy drill sites.[139] The 2 most common sites are the mandibular ramus and symphysis. The author (Bach Le) prefers the mandibular ramus site over the symphysis because of the high postoperative morbidity associated with the latter. Paresthesia, reported to be as high as 52% at 18 months in one study[140] and 22% at 3 years in another,[141] is commonly associated with harvesting from the symphysis. Not only have sensory disturbances been reported, but loss of tooth vitality also has been noted from harvesting bone from the symphysis region. Even when a symphysis graft was harvested beyond the commonly recognized safe distance of 5 mm from the root apices, 33% of teeth still lost vitality.[142] This loss of vitality is likely due to disturbance of the mandibular incisive canal branch of the inferior alveolar nerve.

Success with autogenous block onlay grafts requires adherence to 5 key surgical principles: proper incision design and flap management, adequate recipient site preparation, proper graft adaptation, rigid fixation, and use of particulate graft and membrane.

Proper incision and flap design Proper incision design will facilitate tension-free wound closure, which is especially important when a large volume of graft material is used to overcorrect anatomic defects in anticipation of normal graft shrinkage. The authors prefer the open-book flap because it allows for tension-free closure, rotational advancement of the flap for coronal advancement of the tissue margin, and it is less invasive. Scoring of the periosteum is performed as the last step before particulate graft placement to ensure

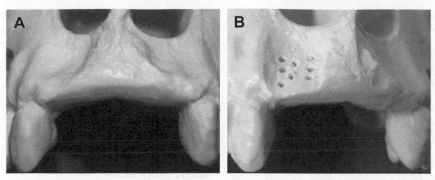

Fig. 14. Recipient site preparation creates more walls to incorporate the graft and promotes RAP. (*A*) Planned recipient site. (*B*) Site preparation. (*Courtesy of* Bach Le, DDS, MD, Los Angeles, CA.)

maximum bleeding for angiogenesis. In addition to scoring the periosteum, it is important to perform split-thickness dissection of the flap to surgically expand the soft tissue matrix to create sufficient space for incorporation of graft material.

Recipient site preparation This involves decorticating the recipient site to create more walls to

incorporate the onlay block graft. Preparing the recipient site also promotes the regional accelerated phenomenon (RAP)[103] to release growth factors and platelets to encourage healing (**Fig. 14**).

Precise graft adaptation Intimate adaptation of the block graft to the prepared recipient site is necessary for graft take (**Fig. 15**A). All sharp edges

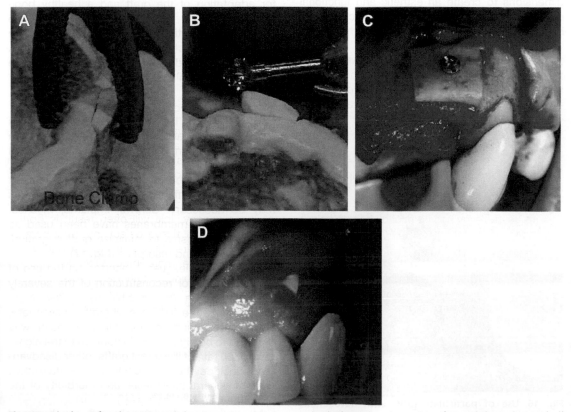

Fig. 15. Block graft adaptation and contouring. Graft must be intimately adapted to the recipient site and all sharp edges removed to prevent tissue dehiscence and partial or total loss of graft. (*A*) Adaptation. (*B*) Contouring. (*C*) Sharp graft edges. (*D*) Graft dehiscence. (*Courtesy of* Bach Le, DDS, MD, Los Angeles, CA.)

should be removed to prevent wound dehiscence and graft exposure (see **Fig. 15**B–D).

Rigid fixation Rigid fixation usually requires 2 screws to prevent rotation of the graft. However, 1 screw is acceptable for small blocks if the graft is rigid.

Particulate graft and bioabsorbable membrane Various bone grafts or bone substitutes have been described for use with and without block grafting for GBR.[82–91] Autogenous onlay block grafts covered with bovine bone have shown to exhibit less resorption.[143] Le and Burstein[95] found that when human mineralized allograft was placed over autogenous block graft and covered with a bioabsorbable membrane, bone and soft tissue contours improved with less need for autogenous bone (**Fig. 16**).

Management of Vertical Defects

Severe vertical alveolar ridge defects are usually 3-dimensional and present a difficult challenge to the implant surgeon. Patients with vertical defects usually have concomitant horizontal defects and these defects must be fully reconstructed in all dimensions to create an esthetic and functional result. Furthermore, many vertical defects usually have loss of bone attachment to the teeth adjacent

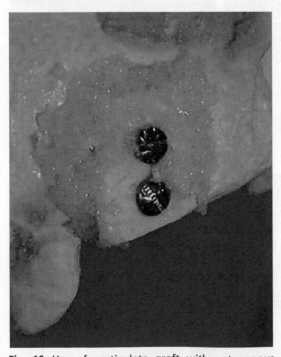

Fig. 16. Use of particulate graft with autogenous block graft. Covering block graft with particulate allograft material. (*Courtesy of* Bach Le, DDS, MD, Los Angeles, CA.)

to the defect. In many instances, it is more beneficial to extract these teeth so that a healthy bone attachment level can be attained for bone grafting.

When a vertical defect is not treated, the patient may require an unaesthetic long clinical crown and/or poor crown-to-root ratio, which may negatively affect the longevity of the implant. These defects may be corrected before or simultaneous with implant placement, depending on the severity of the defect.[76,144–146]

Onlay block bone graft

Autogenous bone graft has long been considered to be the gold standard for grafting severe hard tissue defects. However, reconstruction of large vertical defects often requires a significant amount of autogenous bone, often from extraoral sources. Autogenous block grafts have been described to augment vertical defects, but may be prone to resorption depending on the type of donor bone.[76,113,146,147] It has also been reported that corticocancellous iliac bone is subject to more resorption when the graft site is not prosthetically loaded.[113]

Prerequisites for vertical augmentation using onlay block grafts include a wide recipient bed for adaptation of the graft and a healthy bone attachment level at the teeth adjacent to the grafted span. Vertical augmentation of 3 to 5 mm can usually be achieved using autogenous block grafting. Larger defects may require a 2-stage grafting approach for better outcomes.

Particulate graft

Particulate grafts lack the structural rigidity of an onlay block graft and are subject to graft migration and displacement. Implants can be placed successfully into these grafted sites; however, resorption must be anticipated during treatment planning, as further augmentation procedures may be necessary. Screws, implants, meshes, and reinforced membranes have been used as tenting mechanisms to minimize graft migration, displacement, and resorption (**Fig. 17**).[77,93,94]

Louis and colleagues[93] reported on the use of titanium mesh for reconstruction of the severely atrophic maxilla or mandible using iliac crest bone graft with a 97% overall graft success rate, although exposure of the titanium mesh was reported to be high (52%). In addition to the higher resorption rate of iliac crest grafts, other disadvantages include the high costs of hospitalization, risks of general anesthesia, and morbidity of the procedure.[116,118,119,130]

Mineralized particulate allograft can be used similarly with a tenting mechanism for vertical alveolar ridge augmentation (**Fig. 18**).[77,145,148]

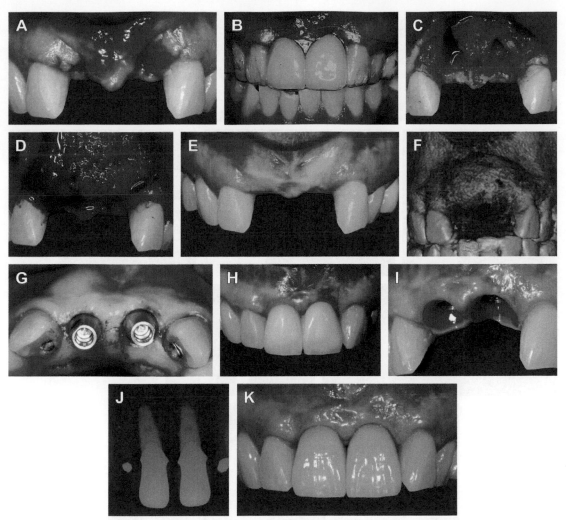

Fig. 17. Particulate grafting for vertical augmentation. Open-book flap design with particulate grafting to correct a vertical defect. (*A*) Preoperative defect. (*B*) Evaluation with Essix. (*C*) Vertical defects. (*D*) Particulate graft. (*E*) Postoperative. (*F*) Bony augmentation. (*G*) Implant replacement. (*H*) Temporary restoration. (*I*) Soft tissue contours. (*J*) Radiograph. (*K*) Final restorations. (*Courtesy of* Bach Le, DDS, MD, Los Angeles, CA.)

Using particulate allograft and screws, an average of 9.2 mm of vertical height was achieved and implants were successfully placed (**Fig. 19**).[145] This technique requires a membrane for optimal results and is technique-sensitive. Vertical defects with large spans (2 missing teeth or more) have a higher risk of wound dehiscence. Correction of these defects in a 2-stage grafting protocol restoring smaller increments per graft may reduce the risk of graft dehiscence. Vertical defects involving a single missing tooth span may be corrected in a 1-staged surgery protocol.[77] When there are failures, it is usually the result of inadequate release of the flap leading to bone graft exposure and resorption. Wound dehiscence can lead to more pronounced bone graft resorption. When using particulate bone, maintaining the soft tissue matrix

is critical. Proper flap design and manipulation is critical to prevent wound dehiscence when using these techniques.

Distraction osteogenesis

Distraction osteogenesis has been described to address the vertically deficient alveolar ridge and is recommended for severe vertical defects (>6–7 mm).[149,150] It is the opinion of the senior author that this technique requires a minimal amount of basal bone width of at least 6 mm to minimize resorption of the transport segment. This technique frequently requires further augmentation procedures depending on the available basal bone and the vector at which the bone is distracted. Although distraction osteogenesis can be a predictable method for vertical augmentation,

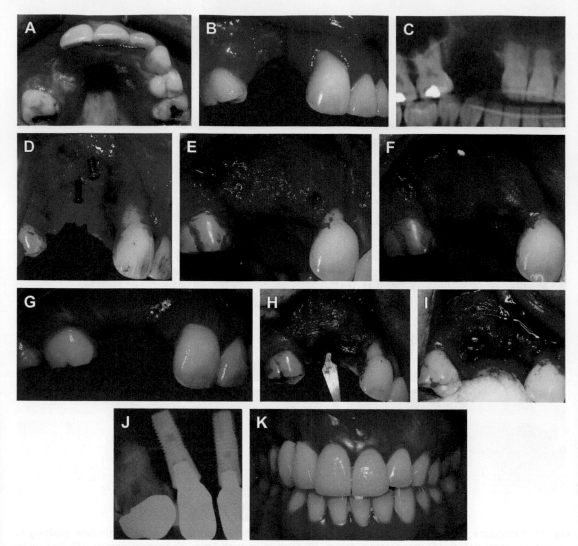

Fig. 18. (*A–K*) Particulate grafting for large vertical defect. Open-book flap design with tenting screws, membrane, and particulate graft to correct a large vertical alveolar defect. (*A*) Large alveolar defect. (*B*) Vertical defect component. (*C*) Radiographic defect. (*D*) Tenting screws. (*E*) Particulate grafting. (*F*) Membrane. (*G*) Postoperative. (*H*) Augmentation result. (*I*) Implant placement. (*J*) Radiograph. (*K*) Final restorations. (*Courtesy of Bach Le, DDS, MD, Los Angeles, CA.*)

complications are common and include lack of buccal augmentation, loss of keratinized tissue, unsatisfactory esthetic result, and a loss of vestibular depth.[151] Furthermore, the success of the technique is highly dependent on patient compliance, and hardware costs will have to be factored into the treatment plan (**Fig. 20**).

Interpositional osteotomy

Interpositional osteotomies can also be used to vertically augment the alveolar ridge.[144,152,153] Moderate to severe vertical defects (between 5 and 6 mm) can be corrected using this technique with minimal resorption around the implants placed into the augmented bone (**Fig. 21**).[153] In

the posterior mandible, transient paresthesia is a common unwanted side effect and 5 mm of basal bone above the inferior alveolar nerve is necessary to carry out this procedure safely without damage to adjacent structures.[152,153]

Laster and colleagues[154] described a similar technique in the premaxilla region using particulate bovine bone matrix as an interpositional graft and used dental implants to fixate the bone segment. Vertical bone height gains averaged 5 mm and required only one surgical procedure because the dental implants were placed simultaneously. Placing dental implants in the correct 3-dimensional position may be difficult with this technique because ideally positioning

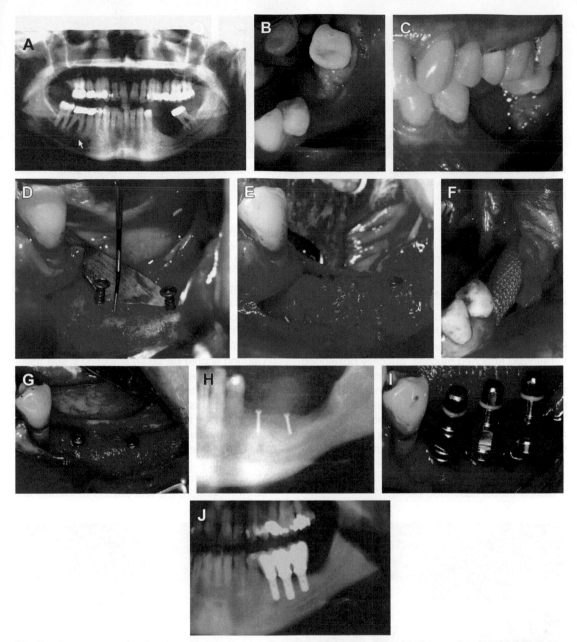

Fig. 19. "Screw tent-pole" (STP) grafting technique for vertical augmentation. (*A–C*) Large localized vertical alveolar ridge defect. (*D,E*) Micro-tenting screws are placed strategically in combination with human mineralized allograft to tent the soft tissue matrix. (*F*) Bioresorbable membrane is placed over the graft material. (*G–I*) Reentry for implant placement at 4 to 5 months after graft placement. (*G*) Augmented bone. (*H*) Radiograph of augmentation. (*I*) Implant placement. (*J*) Final restorations with maintenance of alveolar bone level. (*Courtesy of* Bach Le, DDS, MD, Los Angeles, CA.)

the transported native bone may not be possible. Careful assessment of the alveolar ridge before this procedure and generating a surgical stent may facilitate treatment planning and surgery.

Multiple surgical procedures often are required to achieve an esthetic result when bone augmentation is necessary. At times, a combination of

the previously described techniques may be indicated (eg, onlay block grafting or GBR and distraction osteogenesis). Sometimes an initial augmentation procedure will still not provide sufficient reconstruction of the missing tissue and an additional procedure may be indicated. No matter how many procedures are required, the implant

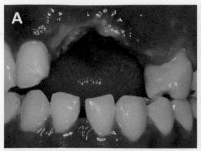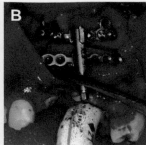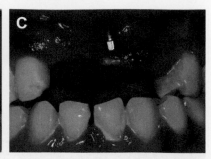

Fig. 20. Alveolar distraction osteogenesis for vertical augmentation. Distraction osteogenesis of a severe vertical bone defect. (*A*) Large vertical defect. (*B*) Alveolar distractor. (*C*) Correction of vertical defect. (*Courtesy of Bach Le, DDS, MD, Los Angeles, CA.*)

surgeon and patient must understand that a natural-appearing result will be difficult to achieve if the bony structure is insufficient.[15]

Soft Tissue Management

Labial recession defects around a dental implant can result in a poor esthetic result. The cause of labial recession is influenced by an inadequate keratinized attached mucosa, buccally positioned implant platform, osseous dehiscence or fenestration, frenal or muscle pull, thin gingival biotype, recurrent inflammation, or iatrogenic factors.[155] To prevent or correct recession defects, soft tissue augmentation may occasionally be required. It is the opinion of the senior author that many dehiscence or recession defects can be corrected by augmentation of the underlying bony defect using a GBR protocol described earlier.[156]

Soft tissue procedures can be used to increase tissue volume, amount of keratinized gingiva, or to improve esthetic outcomes around dental implants.[155,157] However, there is still debate regarding the best techniques for soft tissue manipulation and augmentation. Available soft tissue procedures include pedicle soft tissue grafts, free soft tissue grafts, or a combination of both (**Table 5**).[158–164]

Caution should be taken selecting a soft tissue augmentation technique. Some periodontal procedures used to correct esthetic shortcomings that are successful in natural dentition have occasionally been shown to worsen the esthetic outcome when used between adjacent implants.[15] This is often due to scar contracture of soft tissue grafts causing some recession.

When treatment planning to correct for peri-implant recession, the first step is to identify and

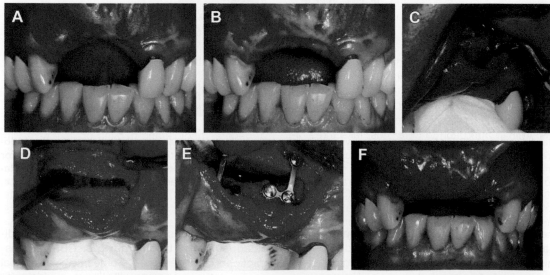

Fig. 21. "Alveolar sandwich graft" (interpositional osteotomy). Initial improvement of severe vertical defect using tenting screws and particulate graft, then secondarily grafted using the "Alveolar sandwich graft" technique. (*A*) Severe vertical defect. (*B*) Reduced defect after initial particulate grafting with tenting screws. (*C*) Osteotomy. (*D*) Mobilized segment. (*E*) Fixated segment. (*F*) Corrected vertical defect. (*Courtesy of Bach Le, DDS, MD, Los Angeles, CA.*)

Table 5 Summary of soft tissue augmentation techniques	
Pedicle Grafts	**Free Grafts**
Rotational Flaps: Lateral sliding flap Oblique rotational flap Transpositioned flap Advanced Flaps: Coronally positioned flap Semilunar coronally positioned flap	Free gingival graft (*epithelialized*) Subepithelial connective tissue graft (*nonepithelialized*)

From Fu JH, Su CY, Wang HL. Esthetic soft tissue management for teeth and implants. J Evid Based Dent Pract 2012;12:129–42; with permission.

correct the cause of the defect.[155] Next, consider the factors that contribute to success for soft tissue augmentation procedures:

- Gingival biotype[165]
- Flap thickness[166]
- Presence of interproximal bone and soft tissue[167]
- Defect dimensions (height, width, and depth)[168]
- Placement of the flap 1 to 2 mm above the cementoenamel junction[166,169]
- Type of augmentation procedure chosen[166,169]

Autogenous grafting

In soft tissue augmentation, autogenous grafting remains the gold standard. The following autogenous grafting techniques have been shown to be effective at increasing keratinized tissue and soft tissue thickness[170]:

- Laterally positioned flap
- Apically positioned flap
- Subepithelial connective tissue graft
- Free gingival grafts

Gains of 1 to 2 mm in soft tissue thickness are possible by using soft tissue augmentation alone.[11]

Alternative grafting options

In addition to autogenous grafting techniques, a variety of alternative options also have been recently tested and shown to be effective.[170] These include the following biological agents and alternative graft materials:

- Freeze-dried skin allografts have been used for keratinized tissue augmentation[155,171]
- Acellular dermal matrix has been used for augmentation of soft tissue thickness and increasing keratinized tissue[172–174]
- Xenogeneic bioabsorbable collagen matrix has been used to increase keratinized tissue[175]
- Guided tissue regeneration using barrier membranes[155]
- Living cellular construct (bilayered cell therapy) for increasing soft tissue thickness and keratinized tissue[155,176,177]
- Biological agents, such as enamel matrix derivative,[178] platelet-rich plasma,[179] and platelet-derived growth factor[155]

Fu and colleagues[155] performed a literature review of the new graft materials available for soft tissue augmentation around dental implants as they compare to autogenous grafting. The findings are reported in **Table 6**.

Implant Position and Angulation

Dental implant therapy is prosthetically driven and not bone-driven. To this end, the implant must be accurately placed in a 3-dimensional (mesiodistal, labiolingual, and apicocoronal) position with the goal of achieving a proper emergence profile for the final restoration.[180] When the implant position

Table 6 Autogenous graft versus xenograft in soft tissue augmentation	
Keratinized tissue gain	Subepithelial connective tissue graft is FAR SUPERIOR to xenogeneic bioabsorbable collagen matrix
Tissue thickness gain	Subepithelial connective tissue graft is SUPERIOR to xenogeneic bioabsorbable collagen matrix
Esthetic outcome	Subepithelial connective tissue graft is SUPERIOR to xenogeneic bioabsorbable collagen matrix

From Fu JH, Su CY, Wang HL. Esthetic soft tissue management for teeth and implants. J Evid Based Dent Pract 2012;12:129–42; with permission.

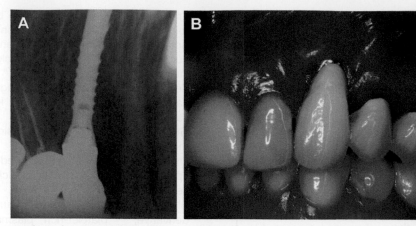

Fig. 22. Deep implant placement (*A*) resulting in unnaturally long restoration (*B*). Implants placed too deep in an apicocoronal position or too labial often result in an unnaturally long restoration. (*Courtesy of* Bach Le, DDS, MD, Los Angeles, CA.)

is not accurate, the esthetic result is often compromised.

The following guidelines assist in achieving ideal implant placement and angulation:

- A minimum of 2 mm of facial bone should be preserved during implant placement[80]
  ○ 6 mm of bone in buccolingual dimension is the minimum amount required for a 3.75-mm–diameter to 4.0-mm–diameter implant
- Allow 1.5 to 2.0 mm of bone between the implant platform and an adjacent tooth
  ○ 5 to 6 mm of bone in the mesiodistal dimension is the minimum amount required for a 3.75-mm–diameter to 4-mm–diameter implant
- Allow 3 mm of bone between adjacent implants[41]
- Implant platform should be located at least 3 mm apical to the ideal gingival margin but no more than 5 mm apical

Implants placed too deep in an apicocoronal position or too labial often result in an unnaturally long restoration (**Fig. 22**). In addition, implant position has been shown to have a direct influence on bone and soft tissue thickness at the implant site.[27]

Le and colleagues[181] studied the relationship between crestal labial soft tissue thickness and implant buccolingual angulation. The buccolingual angulation was recorded as cingulum, incisal, or labial based on the position of the screw access hole on provisional restorations (**Fig. 23**, **Table 7**). The implant labial bone thickness was measured at the crestal and midimplant levels using sectional CBCT scans. Significant differences were detected between crestal labial soft tissue thickness of implants with cingulum and incisal, as well as cingulum and labial angulations (*P*<.01). Of

implants with cingulum, incisal, and labial angulations, 3.4%, 20.0%, and 53.3%, respectively, had a crestal labial soft tissue thickness of less than 2 mm. A significant association between crestal

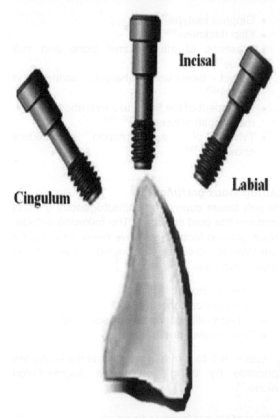

Fig. 23. Implant angulation. (*Courtesy of* Bach Le, DDS, MD, Los Angeles, CA. *From* Le BT, Borzabadi-Farahani A, Pluemsakunthai W. Is buccolingual angulation of maxillary anterior implants associated with the crestal labial soft tissue thickness? Int J Oral Maxillofac Surg 2014;43(7):874–8; with permission.)

Table 7
Implant angulation and crestal labial soft tissue thickness

	Crestal Labial Soft Tissue, mm	
Implant Angulation	**Mean, mm**	**SD**
Labial	1.71	0.72
Incisal	2.24	0.51
Cingulum	2.98	0.84

Significant differences were detected between crestal labial soft tissue thickness of implants with cingulum and incisal, as well as cingulum and labial angulations (P<.01).
From Le BT, Borzabadi-Farahani A, Pluemsakunthai W. Is buccolingual angulation of maxillary anterior implants associated with the crestal labial soft tissue thickness? Int J Oral Maxillofac Surg 2014;43(7):874–8; with permission.

labial soft tissue thickness and implant buccolingual angulation was noted when implant labial bone thickness at crestal level was less than 2 mm (P<.01). Le and colleagues[181] conclude that implants with labial angulations carry a higher risk of soft tissue complications when the crestal implant labial bone thickness is less than 2 mm.

SUMMARY

As the focus in implant dentistry has turned to achieving natural-appearing outcomes, implant survival is no longer considered success. A natural-appearing outcome depends largely on accurate diagnosis and treatment planning, adequate bone and soft tissue augmentation when required, and precise implant position and angulation. The techniques reviewed in this article will allow the implant surgeon to achieve a natural, esthetic outcome.

REFERENCES

1. Ekfeldt A, Carlsson GE, Borjesson G. Clinical evaluation of single-tooth restorations supported by osseointegrated implants: a retrospective study. Int J Oral Maxillofac Surg 1994;9:179–83.
2. Haas R, Mensdorff-Pouilly N, Mailath G, et al. Branemark single tooth implants: a preliminary report of 76 implants. J Prosthet Dent 1995;73:274–9.
3. Jemt T, Laney WR, Harris D, et al. Osseointegrated implants for single tooth replacement: a 1-year report from a multicenter prospective study. Int J Oral Maxillofac Implants 1991;6:29–36.
4. Oates TW, West J, Jones J, et al. Long-term changes in soft tissue height on the facial surface of dental implants. Implant Dent 2002;11:272–9.
5. Tymstra N, Raghoebar GM, Vissink A, et al. Dental implant treatment for two adjacent missing teeth in the maxillary aesthetic zone: a comparative pilot study and test of principle. Clin Oral Implants Res 2011;22:207–13.
6. Belser UC, Grutter L, Vailati F, et al. Outcome evaluation of early placed maxillary anterior single-tooth implants using objective esthetic criteria: a cross-sectional, retrospective study in 45 patients with a 2- to 4-year follow-up using pink and white esthetic scores. J Periodontol 2009;80(1):140–51.
7. Esposito M, Grusovin MG, Worthington HV. Agreement of quantitative subjective evaluation of esthetic changes in implant dentistry by patients and practitioners. Int J Oral Maxillofac Implants 2009;24(2):309–15.
8. Meijndert L, Meijer HJ, Stellingsma K, et al. Evaluation of aesthetics of implant-supported single-tooth replacements using different bone augmentation procedures: a prospective randomized clinical study. Clin Oral Implants Res 2007;18(6):715–9.
9. Kokich VO, Kokich VG, Kiyak HA. Perceptions of dental professionals and laypersons to altered dental esthetics: asymmetric and symmetric situations. Am J Orthod Dentofacial Orthop 2006;130:141–51.
10. Bhuvaneswaran M. Principles of smile design. J Conserv Dent 2010;13:225–32.
11. Palacci P, Nowzari H. Soft tissue enhancement around dental implants. Periodontol 2000 2000;47:113–32.
12. Raj V. Esthetic paradigms in the interdisciplinary management of maxillary anterior dentition–a review. J Esthet Restor Dent 2013;25:295–304.
13. Ward DH. Using the RED proportion to engineer the perfect smile. Dent Today 2008;27:112, 114–112,117.
14. Ward DH. A study of dentists preferred maxillary anterior tooth width proportions: comparing the recurring esthetic dental proportion to other mathematically and naturally occurring proportions. J Esthet Dent 2007;19:338–9.
15. Priest GF. The esthetic challenge of adjacent implants. J Oral Maxillofac Surg 2007;65:2–12.
16. Esposito M, Grusovin MG, Maghaireh H, et al. Interventions for replacing missing teeth: management of soft tissues for dental implants. Cochrane Database Syst Rev 2007;(18):CD006697.
17. Seibert J, Lindhe J. Esthetics and periodontal therapy. In: Lindhe J, editor. Textbook of clinical periodontology. Copenhagen (Denmark): Munksgaard International Publishing; 1989. p. 477–514.
18. De Rouck T, Eghbali R, Collys K, et al. The gingival biotype revisited: transparency of the periodontal probe through the gingival margin as a method to discriminate thin from thick gingiva. J Clin Periodontol 2009;36:428–33.

19. Cosyn J, Eghbali A, De Bruyn H, et al. Single implant treatment in healing versus healed sites of the anterior maxilla: an aesthetic evaluation. Clin Implant Dent Relat Res 2012;14:517–26.

20. Cosyn J, Eghbali A, Hanselaer L, et al. Four modalities of single implant treatment in the anterior maxilla: a clinical, radiographic, and aesthetic evaluation. Clin Implant Dent Relat Res 2013;15:517–30.

21. Eghbali A, De Bruyn H, De Rouck T, et al. Single implant treatment in healing versus healed sites of the anterior maxilla: a clinical and radiographic evaluation. Clin Implant Dent Relat Res 2012;14:336–46.

22. Muller HP, Eger T, Schorb A. Gingival dimensions after root coverage with free connective tissue grafts. J Clin Periodontol 1998;25:424–30.

23. Hammerle CH, Chen ST, Wilson TG. Consensus statements and recommended clinical procedures regarding the placement of implants in extraction sockets. Int J Oral Maxillofac Implants 2004;(19 Suppl):26–8.

24. Chen ST, Darby IB, Reynolds EC, et al. Immediate implant placement postextraction without flap elevation. J Periodontol 2009;80:163–72.

25. Kan JY, Rungcharassaeng K, Morimoto T, et al. Facial gingival tissue stability after connective tissue graft with single immediate tooth replacement in the esthetic zone: consecutive case report. J Oral Maxillofac Surg 2009;67(11 Suppl):40–8.

26. Sclar AG. Preserving alveolar ridge anatomy following tooth removal in conjunction with immediate implant placement. Atlas Oral Maxillofac Surg Clin North Am 1999;7:39–59.

27. Le BT, Borzabadi-Farahani A. Labial bone thickness in area of anterior maxillary implants associated with crestal labial soft tissue thickness. Implant Dent 2012;21(5):406–10.

28. Bengazi F, Wennstrom JL, Lekholm U. Recession of the soft tissue margin at oral implants. A 2-year longitudinal prospective study. Clin Oral Implants Res 1996;7:303–10.

29. Wennstrom JL, Bengazi F, Lekholm U. The influence of the masticatory mucosa on the peri-implant soft tissue condition. Clin Oral Implants Res 1994;5:1–8.

30. Chung DM, Oh TJ, Shotwell JL, et al. Significance of keratinized mucosa in maintenance of dental implants with different surfaces. J Periodontol 2006;77:1410–20.

31. Bouri A Jr, Bissada N, Al-Zahrani MS, et al. Width of keratinized gingiva and the health status of the supporting tissues around dental implants. Int J Oral Maxillofac Implants 2008;23:323–6.

32. Kim BS, Kim YK, Yun PY, et al. Evaluation of peri-implant tissue response according to the presence of keratinized mucosa. Oral Surg Oral Med Oral Pathol Oral Radiol Endod 2009;107:24–8.

33. Cairo F, Pagliaro U, Nieri M. Soft tissue management at implant sites. J Clin Periodontol 2008;35(Suppl 8):163–7.

34. Wennström JL, Derks J. Is there a need for keratinized mucosa around implants to maintain health and tissue stability? Clin Oral Implants Res 2012;23(Suppl 6):136–46.

35. Jung RE, Sailer I, Hämmerle CH, et al. In vitro color changes of soft tissues caused by restorative materials. Int J Periodontics Restorative Dent 2007;27:251–7.

36. Block MS, Mercante DE, Lirette D, et al. Prospective evaluation of immediate and delayed provisional single tooth restorations. J Oral Maxillofac Surg 2009;67(11 Suppl):89–107.

37. Kan JY, Rungcharassaeng K, Umezu K, et al. Dimensions of peri-implant mucosa: an evaluation of maxillary anterior single implants in humans. J Periodontol 2003;74:557–62.

38. Kan JY, Rungcharassaeng K. Interimplant papilla preservation in the esthetic zone: a report of six consecutive cases. Int J Periodontics Restorative Dent 2003;23:249.

39. Botticelli D, Persson LG, Lindhe J, et al. Bone tissue formation adjacent to implants placed in fresh extraction sockets: an experimental study in dogs. Clin Oral Implants Res 2006;17:351.

40. Furhauser R, Florescu D, Benesch T, et al. Evaluation of soft tissue around single-tooth implant crowns: the pink esthetic score. Clin Oral Implants Res 2005;16:639–44.

41. Tarnow D, Elian N, Fletcher P, et al. Vertical distance from the crest of bone to the height of the interproximal papilla between adjacent implants. J Periodontol 2003;74:1785–8.

42. Choquet V, Hermans M, Adriaenssens P, et al. Clinical and radiographic evaluation of the papilla level adjacent to single-tooth dental implants: a retrospective study in the maxillary anterior region. J Periodontol 2001;72:1364–71.

43. Tarnow D, Cho SC, Wallace SS. The effect of interimplant distance on the height of inter-implant bone crest. J Periodontol 2000;71:546–9.

44. De Rouck T, Collys K, Cosyn J. Immediate single-tooth implants in the anterior maxilla: a 1-year case cohort study on hard and soft tissue response. J Clin Periodontol 2008;35:649–57.

45. Kan JY, Rungcharassaeng K, Lozada J. Immediate placement and provisionalization of maxillary anterior single implants: 1-year prospective study. Int J Oral Maxillofac Implants 2003;18:31–9.

46. Kan JY, Rungcharassaeng K, Liddelow G, et al. Periimplant tissue response following immediate provisional restoration of scalloped implants in the esthetic zone: a one-year pilot prospective multicenter study. J Prosthet Dent 2007;97(6 Suppl):S109–18.

47. Salama H, Salama M. The role of orthodontic extrusive remodeling in the enhancement of soft and hard tissue profiles prior to implant placement: a systematic approach to the management of extraction site defects. Int J Periodontics Restorative Dent 1993;13:312–33.

48. Brindis MA, Block MS. Orthodontic tooth extrusion to enhance soft tissue implant esthetics. J Oral Maxillofac Surg 2009;67(11 Suppl):49–59.

49. Hertel RC, Blijdorp PA, Baker DL. A preventive mucosal flap technique for use in implantology. Int J Oral Maxillofac Implants 1993;8:452–8.

50. Lekholm U, Zarb GA. Patient selection and preparation. In: Branemark PI, Zarb GA, Albrektsson T, editors. Osseointegration in clinical dentistry. Chicago: Quintessence; 1985. p. 199–209.

51. Norton MR, Gamble C. Bone classification: an objective scale of bone density using the computerized tomography scan. Clin Oral Implants Res 2001;12:79–84.

52. Ono Y, Nevins M, Cappett EG. The need for keratinized tissue for implants. In: Nevins M, Mellonig JT, editors. Implant therapy. Clinical approaches and evidence of success 2003;2. (IL): Quintessence Publishing Co, Inc; p. 227–37.

53. Schropp L, Wenzel A, Kostopoulos L, et al. Bone healing and soft tissue contour changes following single-tooth extraction: a clinical and radiographic 12-month prospective study. Int J Periodontics Restorative Dent 2003;23:313–23.

54. Pietrokovski J, Massler M. Alveolar ridge resorption following tooth extraction. J Prosthet Dent 1967;17:21–7.

55. Araujo M, Lindhe J. Dimensional ridge alterations following tooth extraction. An experimental study in the dog. J Clin Periodontol 2005;32:212–8.

56. Bidra AS, Rungruanganunt P. Omega-Shaped (Ω) incision design to enhance gingival esthetics for adjacent implant placement in the anterior region. J Oral Maxillofac Surg 2011;69:2144–51.

57. Pradeep AR, Karthikeyan BV. Peri-implant papilla reconstruction: realities and limitations. J Periodontol 2006;77:534.

58. Atwood DA, Coy WA. Clinical, cephalometric, and densitometric study of reduction of residual ridges. J Prosthet Dent 1971;26:280.

59. Barone A, Aldini NN, Fini M, et al. Xenograft versus extraction alone for ridge preservation after tooth removal: a clinical and histomorphometric study. J Periodontol 2008;79:1370–7.

60. Lekovic V, Kenney EB, Weinlaender M, et al. A bone regenerative approach to alveolar ridge maintenance following tooth extraction. Report of 10 cases. J Periodontol 1997;68:563–70.

61. Artzi Z, Tal H, Dayan D. Porous bovine bone mineral in healing of human extraction sockets. Part 1: histomorphometric evaluations at 9 months. J Periodontol 2000;71:1015–23.

62. Iasella JM, Greenwell H, Miller RL, et al. Ridge preservation with freeze-dried allograft and a collagen membrane compared to extraction alone for implant site development: a clinical and histologic study in humans. J Periodontol 2003;73:990–9.

63. Fickl S, Zuhr O, Wachtel H, et al. Dimensional changes of the alveolar ridge contour after different socket preservation techniques. J Clin Periodontol 2008;35:906–13.

64. Kan J, Rungcharassaeng K, Sclar A, et al. Effects of facial osseous defect morphology on gingival dynamics after immediate tooth replacement and guided bone regeneration: 1-year results. J Oral Maxillofac Surg 2007;65(7 Suppl 1):13–9.

65. De Sanctis M, Vignoletti F, Discepoli N, et al. Immediate implants at fresh extraction sockets: bone healing in four different implant systems. J Clin Periodontol 2009;36:705–11.

66. Covani U, Cornelini R, Barone A. Vertical crestal bone changes around implants placed into fresh extraction sockets. J Periodontol 2007;78:810–5.

67. Botticelli D, Berglundh T, Lindhe J. Hard-tissue alterations following immediate implant placement in extraction sites. J Clin Periodontol 2004;31:820–8.

68. Evans CD, Chen ST. Esthetic outcomes of immediate implant placements. Clin Oral Implants Res 2008;19:73–80.

69. Grunder U, Gracis S, Capelli M. Influence of the 3-D bone-to-implant relationship on esthetics. Int J Periodontics Restorative Dent 2005;25:113.

70. Favero G, Lang NP, Leon IG, et al. Role of teeth adjacent to implants installed immediately into extraction sockets: an experimental study in the dog. Clin Oral Implants Res 2012;23(4):402–8.

71. Le B, Burstein J. Esthetic grafting for small volume hard and soft tissue contour defects for implant site development. Implant Dent 2008;17:136–41.

72. Belser UC, Schmid B, Higginbottom F, et al. Outcome analysis of implant restorations located in the anterior maxilla: a review of the recent literature. Int J Oral Maxillofac Implants 2004;19:30.

73. Schenk RK, Buser D, Hardwick WR, et al. Healing pattern of bone regeneration in membrane-protected defects: a histologic study in the canine mandible. Int J Oral Maxillofac Implants 1994;9:13–29.

74. Sculean A, Nikolidakis D, Schwarz F. Regeneration of periodontal tissues: combinations of barrier membranes and grafting materials-biological foundation and preclinical evidence: a systematic review. J Clin Periodontol 2008;35(Suppl 8):106–16.

75. Tolstunov L. Maxillary tuberosity block bone graft: innovative technique and case report. J Oral Maxillofac Surg 2009;67:1723–9.

76. Roccuzzo M, Ramieri G, Spada MC, et al. Vertical alveolar ridge augmentation by means of a titanium mesh and autogenous bone grafts. Clin Oral Implants Res 2004;15:73–81.

77. Le BT, Rohrer MD, Prassad HS. Screw "tent-pole" grafting technique for reconstruction of large vertical alveolar ridge defects using human mineralized allograft for implant site preparation. J Oral Maxillofac Surg 2010;68:428–35.

78. Jensen OT, Cockrell R, Kuhike L, et al. Anterior maxillary alveolar distraction osteogenesis: a prospective 5-year clinical study. Int J Oral Maxillofac Implants 2002;17:52.

79. Jensen OT. Segmental alveolar split combined with dental extractions and osteotome sinus floor intrusion in posterior maxilla using BMP-2/ACS allograft for alveolar reconstruction: technical note and report of three cases. J Oral Maxillofac Surg 2014;71:2040–7.

80. Spray JR, Black CG, Morris HF, et al. The influence of bone thickness on facial marginal bone response: stage 1 placement through stage 2 uncovering. Ann Periodontol 2000;5:119–28.

81. Takahashi T, Fukuda M, Yamaguchi T, et al. Use of endosseous implants for dental reconstruction of patients with grafted alveolar clefts. J Oral Maxillofac Surg 1997;66:251–5.

82. Howell TH, Fiorellini J, Jones A, et al. A feasibility study evaluating rhBMP-2/absorbable collagen sponge device for local alveolar ridge preservation or augmentation. Int J Periodontics Restorative Dent 1997;17:124–39.

83. Buser D, Dula K, Hirt HP, et al. Lateral ridge augmentation using autografts and barrier membranes: a clinical study with 40 partially edentulous patients. J Oral Maxillofac Surg 1996;54:420–32.

84. Hasson O. Lateral ridge augmentation using the pocket technique. J Oral Maxillofac Surg 2005; 63(Suppl 1):26–7.

85. Peleg M. Lateral alveolar ridge augmentation with allogeneic block grafts: observations form a multicenter prospective clinical trial. J Oral Maxillofac Surg 2005;63(Suppl 1):29.

86. Block M, Degen M. Horizontal ridge augmentation using human mineralized particulate bone: preliminary results. J Oral Maxillofac Surg 2004; 62:67–72.

87. Raghoebar GM, Batenburg RH, Vissink A, et al. Augmentation of localized defects of the anterior maxillary ridge with autogenous bone before insertion of implants. J Oral Maxillofac Surg 1996;54: 1180–5.

88. Barone A, Varanini P, Orlando B, et al. Deep-frozen allogeneic onlay bone grafts for reconstruction of atrophic maxillary alveolar ridges: a preliminary study. J Oral Maxillofac Surg 2009;67:1300–6.

89. Oda T, Suzuki H, Yokota M, et al. Horizontal alveolar distraction of the narrow maxilla ridge for implant placement. J Oral Maxillofac Surg 2004; 62:1530–4.

90. Donovan MG, Dickerson NC, Hanson LJ, et al. Maxillary and mandibular reconstruction using calvarial bone grafts and Branemark implants: a preliminary report. J Oral Maxillofac Surg 1994;52: 588–94.

91. Peleg M, Garg AK, Misch CM, et al. Maxillary sinus and ridge augmentations using a surface-derived autogenous bone graft. J Oral Maxillofac Surg 2004;62:1535–44.

92. Llambes F, Silvestre FJ, Caffesse R. Vertical guided bone regeneration with bioabsorbably barrier. J Periodontol 2007;78:2036–42.

93. Louis PJ, Gutta R, Said-Al-Naief N, et al. Reconstruction of the maxilla and mandible with particulate bone graft and titanium mesh for implant placement. J Oral Maxillofac Surg 2008;66:235–45.

94. Marx RE, Shellenberger T, Wimsatt J, et al. Severely resorbed mandible: predictable reconstruction with soft tissue matrix expansion (tent pole) grafts. J Oral Maxillofac Surg 2002;60: 878–88.

95. Le B, Burstein J. Cortical tenting grafting technique in the severely atrophic alveolar ridge for implant site preparation. Implant Dent 2008;17:40–50.

96. Verdugo F, Simonian K, Nowzari H. Periodontal biotype influence on the volume maintenance of only grafts. J Periodontol 2009;80:816–23.

97. Le BT. Effectiveness of single-staged implant placement with simultaneous grafting using mineralized allograft. J Oral Maxillofac Surg 2009; 67(Suppl 1):57.

98. Hellem S, Astrand P, Stenström B, et al. Implant treatment in combination with lateral augmentation of the alveolar process: a 3-year prospective study. Clin Implant Dent Relat Res 2003;5:233–40.

99. Becker W, Dahlin C, Becker B, et al. The use of e-PTFE barrier membranes for bone promotion around titanium implants placed into extraction sockets: a prospective multicenter study. Int J Oral Maxillofac Implants 1994;9:31–40.

100. Buser D, Ruskin J, Higginbotton F, et al. Osseointegration of titanium implants in bone regenerated in membrane-protected defects: a histologic study in the canine mandible. Int J Oral Maxillofac Implants 1995;10:666–81.

101. Dahlin C, Gottlow J, Linde A, et al. Healing of maxillary and mandibular defects using a membrane technique. An experimental study in monkeys. Scand J Plast Reconstr Surg Hand Surg 1990; 24:13–9.

102. Mellonig J, Nevins M, Sanchez R. Evaluation of a bioabsorbable physical barrier for guided bone

regeneration. Part II. Material and a bone replacement graft. Int J Periodontics Restorative Dent 1998;18:139–49.

103. Frost HM. The regional acceleratory phenomenon: a review. Henry Ford Hosp Med J 1983;31:3–9.

104. Araujo MJ, Sonohara M, Hayacibara R, et al. Lateral ridge augmentation by the use of grafts comprised of autologous bone or biomaterial. An experiment in the dog. J Clin Periodontol 2002; 29:1122–31.

105. Le BT, Borzabadi-Farahani A. Simultaneous implant placement and bone grafting with particulate mineralized allograft in sites with buccal wall defects, a three-year follow-up and review of literature. J Craniomaxillofac Surg 2014;42(5): 552–9.

106. Jensen SS, Bosshardt DD, Gruber R, et al. Long-term stability of contour augmentation in the esthetic zone. Histologic and histomorphometric evaluation of 12 human biopsies 14 to 80 months after augmentation. J Periodontol 2014;10:1–15.

107. Karlsen K. Gingival reactions to dental restorations. Acta Odontol Scand 1970;28:895–904.

108. Wang HL, Boyapati L. "PASS" principles for predictable bone regeneration. Implant Dent 2006;15:8.

109. Elian N, Cho SC, Froum S, et al. A simplified socket classification and repair technique. Pract Proced Aesthet Dent 2007;19:99.

110. Covani U, Cornelini R, Barone A. Buccal bone augmentation around immediate implants with and without flap elevation: a modified approach. Int J Oral Maxillofac Implants 2008;23:841.

111. Nishimura I, Shimizu Y, Ooya K. Effects of cortical bone perforation on experimental guided bone regeneration. Clin Oral Implants Res 2004;15:293–300.

112. Slotte C, Lundgren D, Sennerby L, et al. Surgical intervention in enchondral and membranous bone: intraindividual comparisons in the rabbit. Clin Implant Dent Relat Res 2003;5:263–8.

113. Keller EE, Tolman DE, Eckert S. Surgical-prosthodontic reconstruction of advanced maxillary bone compromise with autogenous onlay block grafts and osseointegrated implants: a 12 year study of 32 consecutive patients. Int J Oral Maxillofac Implants 1999;14:197–209.

114. Buser D, Dula K, Belser UC, et al. Localized ridge augmentation using guided bone regeneration. II. Surgical procedure in the mandible. Int J Periodontics Restorative Dent 1995;15:11–29.

115. Buser D, Dula K, Hess D, et al. Localized ridge augmentation with autografts and barrier membranes. Periodontol 2000 1999;19:151–63.

116. Misch CM. Comparison of intraoral donor sites for onlay grafting prior to implant placement. Int J Oral Maxillofac Implants 1997;12:767–76.

117. Rasmusson L, Meredith N, Kahnberg KE, et al. Effects of barrier membranes on bone resorption and implant stability in onlay bone grafts. An experimental study. Clin Oral Implants Res 1999;10: 267–77.

118. Proussaefs P, Lozada J, Rohrer MD. A clinical and histologic evaluation of a block onlay graft in conjunction with autogenous particulate and inorganic bovine material: a case report. Int J Periodontics Restorative Dent 2002;22:567–73.

119. Misch CM, Misch CE. The repair of localized severe ridge defects for implant placement using mandibular bone grafts. Implant Dent 1995;4: 261–7.

120. Thor A. Reconstruction of the anterior maxilla with platelet gel, autogenous bone and titanium mesh: a case report. Clin Implant Dent Relat Res 2002; 4:150–5.

121. Doblin JM, Salkin LM, Mellado JR, et al. A histologic evaluation of localized ridge augmentation utilizing DFDBA in combination with e-PTFE membranes and stainless steel bone pins in humans. Int J Periodontics Restorative Dent 1996; 16:121–9.

122. Fugazzotto PA. Report of 302 consecutive ridge augmentation procedures: technical considerations and clinical results. Int J Oral Maxillofac Implants 1998;13:358–68.

123. Friedmann A, Strietzel FP, Maretzki B, et al. Histological assessment of augmented jaw bone utilizing a new collagen barrier membrane compared to a standard barrier membrane to protect granular bone substitute material: a randomized clinical trial. Clin Oral Implants Res 2002;13:587–94.

124. Kent JN, Quinn JH, Zide MF, et al. Alveolar ridge augmentation using nonresorbable hydroxyapatite with or without autogenous cancellous bone. J Oral Maxillofac Surg 1983;41:629–42.

125. Mentag PJ, Kosinski T. Hydroxyapatite-augmented sites as receptors for replacement implants. J Oral Implantol 1989;15:114–23.

126. Nowzari H, Aalam AA. Mandibular cortical bone graft part 2: surgical technique, applications, and morbidity. Compend Contin Educ Dent 2007;28: 274–80.

127. Aalam AA, Nowzari H. Mandibular cortical bone grafts part 1: anatomy, healing process, and influencing factors. Compend Contin Educ Dent 2007; 28:206–12.

128. Smith JD, Abramson M. Membranous vs. endochondral bone autografts. Arch Otolaryngol 1974; 99:203–5.

129. Zins JE, Whitaker LA. Membranous vs endochondral bone autografts: implications for craniofacial reconstruction. Plast Reconstr Surg 1983;72: 778–85.

130. James JD, Geist ET, Gross BD. Adynamic ileus as a complication of iliac bone removal. J Oral Maxillofac Surg 1981;39:289–91.

131. Proussaefs P, Lozada J, Kleinman A, et al. The use of ramus autogenous block grafts for vertical alveolar ridge augmentation and implant placement: a pilot study. Int J Oral Maxillofac Implants 2002;17:238–48.

132. Montazem A, Valauri DV, St-Hilaire H, et al. The mandibular symphysis as a donor site in maxillofacial bone grafting: a quantitative anatomic study. J Oral Maxillofac Surg 2000;58:1368–71.

133. Gungormus M, Yavuz MS. The ascending ramus of the mandible as a donor site in maxillofacial bone grafting. J Oral Maxillofac Surg 2002;60:1316–8.

134. Misch CM. Ridge augmentation using mandibular ramus bone grafts for the placement of dental implants: presentation of a technique. Pract Periodontics Aesthet Dent 1996;8:127.

135. Pikos MA. Facilitating implant placement with chin graft as donor sites for maxillary bone augmentation. Dent Implantol Update 1995;6:89.

136. Widmark G, Andersson B, Ivanoff CJ. Mandibular bone graft in the anterior maxilla for single-tooth implants: presentation of a surgical method. Int J Oral Maxillofac Surg 1997;26:106–9.

137. Raghoebar GM, Timmenga NM, Reintsema H, et al. Maxillary bone grafting for insertion of endosseous implants: results after 12–124 months. Clin Oral Implants Res 2001;12:279.

138. Proussaefs P. Clinical and histologic evaluation of the use of mandibular tori as donor site for mandibular block grafts: report of three cases. Int J Periodontics Restorative Dent 2006;26:43.

139. Hassani A, Motamedi MH, Tabeshfar S, et al. The "crescent" graft: a new design for bone reconstruction in implant dentistry. J Oral Maxillofac Surg 2009;67:1735–8.

140. Clavero J, Lundgren S. Ramus or chin grafts for maxillary sinus inlay and local onlay augmentation: comparison of donor site morbidity and complications. Clin Implant Dent Relat Res 2003;5:154–60.

141. Weibull L, Widmark G, Ivanoff CJ, et al. Morbidity after chin bone harvesting–a retrospective long-term follow-up study. Clin Implant Dent Relat Res 2009;11:149–57.

142. Sbordone L, Menchini-Fabris GB, Toti P, et al. Clinical survey of neurosensory side-effects of mandibular parasymphyseal bone harvesting. Int J Oral Maxillofac Surg 2009;38:139–45.

143. Maiorana C, Beretta M, Salina S, et al. Reduction of autogenous bone graft resorption by means of bio-oss coverage: a prospective study. Int J Peridontics Restorative Dent 2005;25:19–25.

144. Block M, Haggerty C. Interpositional osteotomy for posterior mandible ridge augmentation. J Oral Maxillofac Surg 2009;67:31–9.

145. Hearne J, Le BT. Screw "tent-pole" grafting technique for vertical augmentation of the severely atrophic alveolar ridge for implant site preparation. J Oral Maxillofac Surg 2008;66(Suppl 1):86–7.

146. Roccuzzo M, Ramieri G, Bunino M, et al. Autogenous bone graft alone or associated with titanium mesh for vertical alveolar ridge augmentation: a controlled clinical trial. Clin Oral Implants Res 2007;18:286–94.

147. Polini F, Robiony M, Sembronio S, et al. Bifunctional sculpturing of the bone graft for 3-dimensional augmentation of the atrophic posterior mandible. J Oral Maxillofac Surg 2009;67:174–7.

148. Fontana F, Santoro F, Maiorana C, et al. Clinical and histologic evaluation of allogeneic bone matrix versus autogenous bone chips associated with titanium-reinforced e-PTFE membrane for vertical ridge augmentation: a prospective pilot study. Int J Oral Maxillofac Implants 2008;23:1003–12.

149. Klug CN, Millesi-Schobel GA, Millesi W, et al. Preprosthetic vertical distraction osteogenesis of the mandible using an L-shaped osteotomy and titanium membranes for guided bone regeneration. J Oral Maxillofac Surg 2001;59:1302–8.

150. Block MS, Baughman DG. Reconstruction of severe maxillary defects using distraction osteogenesis, bone grafts, and implants. J Oral Maxillofac Surg 2005;63:291–7.

151. Froum SJ, Rosenberg ES, Elian N, et al. Distraction osteogenesis for ridge augmentation: prevention and treatment of complications. Thirty case reports. Int J Periodontics Restorative Dent 2008;28:337–45.

152. Jensen OT. Alveolar segmental "sandwich" osteotomies for posterior edentulous mandibular sites for dental implants. J Oral Maxillofac Surg 2006;64:471–5.

153. Jensen OT. Alveolar segmental sandwich osteotomy for anterior maxillary vertical augmentation prior to implant placement. J Oral Maxillofac Surg 2006;64:290–6.

154. Laster Z, Cohen G, Nagler R. A novel technique for vertical bone augmentation in the premaxillary region. J Oral Maxillofac Surg 2009;67:2669–72.

155. Fu JH, Su CY, Wang HL. Esthetic soft tissue management for teeth and implants. J Evid Based Dent Pract 2012;12:129–42.

156. Le BT, Borzabadi-Farahani A, Nielsen B. Management of the ailing implant: an innovative technique for the treatment of labial gingival recession around dental implants [Abstract]. Dental Implant Abstract/How I Do It Session; AAOMS 2014.

157. Israelson H, Plemons JM. Dental implants, regenerative techniques, and periodontal plastic surgery to restore maxillary anterior esthetics. Int J Oral Maxillofac Implants 1993;8:555–61.

158. Harvey PM. Management of advanced periodontitis. I. Preliminary report of a method of surgical reconstruction. N Z Dent J 1965;61(285):180–7.

159. Tarnow DP. Semilunar coronally repositioned flap. J Clin Periodontol 1986;13(3):182–5.

160. Grupe HE, Warren R. Repair of gingival defects by a sliding flap operation. J Periodontol 1956;27:92.

161. Cohen DW, Ross SE. The double papillae repositioned flap in periodontal therapy. J Periodontol 1968;39(2):65–70.

162. Pennel BM, Higgason JD, Towner JD, et al. Oblique rotated flap. J Periodontol 1965;36:305–9.

163. Sullivan HC, Atkins JH. Free autogenous gingival grafts. 3. Utilization of grafts in the treatment of gingival recession. Periodontics 1968;6(4):152–60.

164. Langer B, Langer L. Subepithelial connective tissue graft technique for root coverage. J Periodontol 1985;56(12):715–20.

165. Kao RT, Pasquinelli K. Thick vs thin gingival tissue: a key determinant in tissue response to disease and restorative treatment. J Calif Dent Assoc 2002;30(7):521–6.

166. Huang LH, Neiva RE, Wang HL. Factors affecting the outcomes of coronally advanced flap root coverage procedure. J Periodontol 2005;76(10):1729–34.

167. Miller MB. Aesthetic anterior reconstruction using a combined periodontal/restorative approach. Pract Periodontics Aesthet Dent 1993;5:33–40.

168. Chambrone L, Pannuti CM, Tu YK, et al. Evidence-based periodontal plastic surgery. II. An individual data meta-analysis for evaluating factors in achieving complete root coverage. J Periodontol 2012;83(4):477–90.

169. Pini Prato GP, Clauser C, Cortellini P. Periodontal plastic and mucogingival surgery. Periodontol 2000 1995;2000(9):90–105.

170. Leong DJ, Wang HL. A decision tree for soft tissue grafting. Int J Periodontics Restorative Dent 2011;31(3):307–13.

171. Yukna RA, Sullivan WM. Evaluation of resultant tissue type following the intraoral transplantation of various lyophilized soft tissues. J Periodontal Res 1978;13(2):177–84.

172. Saadoun AP. Root coverage with Emdogain/AlloDerm: a new way to treat gingival recessions. Eur J Esthet Dent 2008;3(1):46–65.

173. Park SH, Wang HL. Management of localized buccal dehiscence defect with allografts and acellular dermal matrix. Int J Periodontics Restorative Dent 2006;26(6):589–95.

174. Park JB. Increasing the width of keratinized mucosa around endosseous implant using acellular dermal matrix allograft. Implant Dent 2006;15(3):275–81.

175. Lorenzo R, Garcia V, Orsini M, et al. Clinical efficacy of a xenogeneic collagen matrix in augmenting keratinized mucosa around implants: a randomized controlled prospective clinical trial. Clin Oral Implants Res 2012;23(3):316–24.

176. Wilson TG Jr, McGuire MK, Nunn ME. Evaluation of the safety and efficacy of periodontal applications of a living tissue-engineered human fibroblast-derived dermal substitute. II. Comparison to the subepithelial connective tissue graft: a randomized controlled feasibility study. J Periodontol 2005;76(6):881–9.

177. McGuire MK, Nunn ME. Evaluation of the safety and efficacy of periodontal applications of a living tissue-engineered human fibroblast-derived dermal substitute. I. Comparison to the gingival autograft: a randomized controlled pilot study. J Periodontol 2005;76(6):867–80.

178. Sculean A, Schwarz F, Becker J, et al. The application of an enamel matrix protein derivative (Emdogain) in regenerative periodontal therapy: a review. Med Princ Pract 2007;16(3):167–80.

179. Petrungaro PS. Using platelet-rich plasma to accelerate soft tissue maturation in esthetic periodontal surgery. Compend Contin Educ Dent 2001;22(9):729–32, 734, 736. [quiz: 746].

180. Kinsel RP, Lamb RE. Tissue-directed placement of dental implants in the esthetic zone for long-term biologic synergy: a clinical report. Int J Oral Maxillofac Implants 2005;20:913.

181. Le BT, Borzabadi-Farahani A, Pluemsakunthai W. Is buccolingual angulation of maxillary anterior implants associated with the crestal labial soft tissue thickness? Int J Oral Maxillofac Surg 2014;43(7):874–8.

Hard and Soft Tissue Surgical Complications in Dental Implantology

Shahid R. Aziz, DMD, MD

KEYWORDS

- Hard tissue • Soft tissue • Implant • Complications • Nerve injury • Peri-implantitis

KEY POINTS

- Complications can be avoided with proper surgical technique and treatment planning.
- Soft tissue complications include nerve injury, flapless surgical complications, and sinus complications.
- Hard tissue complications include complications from bone grafting and peri-implantitis.

No matter what measures are taken, doctors will sometimes falter, and it isn't reasonable to ask that we achieve perfection. What is reasonable is to ask (is) that we never cease to aim for it.
—*Atul Gawande, Complications: A Surgeon's Notes on an Imperfect Science*

INTRODUCTION

As with all surgical procedures, complications will occur. One can expect that the longer one is in surgical practice, the more procedures performed, there will be complications. Dental implantology is no different. The purpose of this article is to discuss surgical complications associated with the placement of dental implants, specifically focusing on how they occur (etiology), as well as their management and prevention. Dental implant surgical complications can be classified into those of hard and soft tissues.

Soft Tissue Complications

Mandibular nerve injury

The third branch of the trigeminal nerve (mandibular nerve or inferior alveolar nerve, IAN) is at constant risk of injury secondary to any mandibular oral and maxillofacial surgical procedure. This nerve provides sensation to the lower lip and chin, as well as innervating the associated dentition. It also provides motor innervation for the muscles of mastication and sensation to the tongue. Injury to the IAN can result in partial or complete paresthesia, analgesia, anesthesia, or in rare cases dysesthesia, to the structures it innervates.[1] The incidence of IAN injury secondary to dental implant surgery is variable, with a range of 0% to 44% in the literature.[2] The etiology of IAN injury is usually associated with inadequate planning or overzealous implant placement, with injury occurring as a result of either miscalculation of nerve position from the preoperative radiographic assessment or injury via placing implant drills or fixture too apical into the nerve canal. In rare cases, the IAN can be injured from local anesthetic injection (injection injury) or retraction of the gingival flap causing stretching of the mental nerve (terminal branch of the IAN). In the edentulous/atrophic mandible, the mental foramen may be located at the crest of the alveolar ridge, and it can be at a higher risk of being traumatized from incision and flap elevation. Prevention of IAN injury is directly related to proper and thorough preoperative implant planning.

Department of Oral and Maxillofacial Surgery, Rutgers School of Dental Medicine, 110 Bergen Street, Room B854, Newark, NJ 07103, USA
E-mail address: azizsr@sdm.rutgers.edu

Oral Maxillofacial Surg Clin N Am 27 (2015) 313–318
http://dx.doi.org/10.1016/j.coms.2015.01.006

Ideally Cone beam computerized tomograms (CBCTs) or conventional computed tomography (CT) scans can be utilized as part of the treatment planning phase to not only plan for implant size, location, and vector of placement, but also to identify and avoid the mandibular canal. Proper measurements and the use of implant planning software are all excellent tools in planning ideal implant placement that avoids injury to the IAN. If a panoramic radiograph is used, the surgeon must be able to adequately visualize the course of the IAN in the mandibular body and para-symphysis regions. When measuring the distance of the alveolar ridge to mandibular nerve canal, one must factor in up to a 25% magnification (magnification factor of 1.25) on the panoramic radiograph. As such, clinical bone height can be more adequately planned by dividing radiographic bone height by the magnification factor (usually 1.25) according to the formula:

Clinical bone height = radiographic bone height/ magnification factor

For example, if the measured radiographic bone height is 13 mm, dividing by 1.25 gives a clinical measurement of 10.4 mm, then the use of an implant fixture less than 10.4 mm will ensure that the IAN will be protected.

Intraoperatively, utilizing CT-based surgical guides (presurgically fabricated based on CT evaluation during the treatment planning phase with precise CT-based placement of the dental implant with depth control away from IAN) can also protect the IAN. Other options include taking radiographs step by step during the procedure with either a drill or positioning locator in place to ensure that the drilling has not gone more apical than planned. If radiographically the IAN canal is violated or it appears that a drill has gone too apical, options include using shorter drills for a shorter implant, aborting the procedure with or without a bone graft, or

redirecting fixture placement. If the radiograph indicates that the canal is violated, clinical assessment can give clues to extent of injury (if any). Violation or injury to the IAN will cause electric shock like pain in even those with good nerve block; the appearance of significant (though transient) bleeding may occur out of osteotomy. Use of local infiltatration as opposed to nerve block can also maintain patient feedback while drilling in the posterior mandible. Topical dexamethasone has been suggested to reduce inflammation in the site of injury. If there is witnessed gross injury to the mandibular canal or IAN, then immediate referral to a microsurgery specialist for treatment is indicated.

An immediate postoperative panoramic radiograph must be taken to assess the placement of the implant(s). If the IAN canal appears encroached, the implant must be backed out or removed. If the implant appears positioned clear of the canal, but the patient has a consistent paresthesia that has not improved within 2 to 3 days after surgery, it is reasonable to either observe or obtain a CBCT to assess if the canal was damaged during placement. If there appears to be damage to the canal (most likely from overzealous drilling) referral to a microsurgery specialist is indicated. If there is no injury to the canal, but the paresthesia persists and the implant appears close to the canal, backing out or removing the implant is indicated. If there does not appear to be encroachment of the implant on or injury to the mandibular canal, postoperative edema maybe the cause of the paresthesia, and a course of corticosteroids may be helpful. If there appears to be no improvement, then consideration of an injection injury must be considered and referral to a microsurgery specialist (**Fig. 1**).

Sinus/nasal floor perforation

Perforation of the maxillary sinus and nasal floor occur, usually secondary to poor planning or

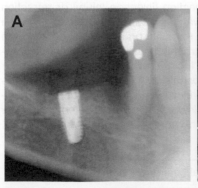
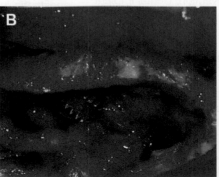
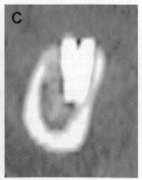

Fig. 1. (*A*) Panoramic radiograph of implant placed into right mandibular canal. (*B*) Buccal plate bone window created with implant into mandibular canal and neurovascular bundle. (*C*) Coronal CT scan with implant into canal. (*Courtesy of* Dr Vincent Ziccardi, Newark, NJ.)

surgical technique. However, in both cases, the degree of perforation dictates treatment. If the perforation occurs with the pilot drill and is minor, often shortening the length of the subsequent osteotomies is enough to avoid significant damage to the underlying membrane. Larger perforations may be treated via internal sinus lifts or placing collagen membrane or infusing rhBMP graft (Medtronic, Minneapolis, Minnesota) at the apex of the osteotomy. In the situation of large perforations, abortion of the placement of the implant is required, replaced with collagen membrane placement at the apex of the osteotomy with bone grafting to avoid sinus complications. Nasal floor perforations may be associated with minor nasal bleeding, which is often transient. In both situations, sinus precautions postoperatively, as well as appropriate antibiotic coverage, is indicated. Displacement of the implant into the maxillary sinus demands immediate foreign body removal. If unable to remove through the existing implant osteotomy, a Caldwell-Luc approach is indicated for retrieval of a displaced implant. Sinus precautions (antibiotics with sinus flora coverage and decongestants) are indicated for 7 to 10 days after the procedure (**Fig. 2**).

Flapless surgery complications

The flapless surgical technique is designed to minimize surgical bleeding and postoperative discomfort. Placement typically utilizes a tissue punch to remove gingiva in the area of implant placement. A major disadvantage of this technique is not being able to fully appreciate the anatomy of the alveolar bone. This is a blind surgical technique; perforation of the buccal or lingual/palatal cortices may occur without the surgeon's knowledge, compromising the fixture. Further, the inability to visualize the crestal bone may result in implants that are too shallow or placed too deep, creating prosthetic problems. Prevention of these

complications is primarily through proper patient selection and good implant treatment planning. Preoperative CBCT with virtual surgical planning for implant placement is often indicated. Assessment of the alveolar width of the ridge and associated curvature can be done via a CBCT. A virtual surgically planned implant guide can eliminate many of these problems as well as ensure placement of the implant into the presurgically determined ideal position and depth. Plain dental radiographs immediately following implant placement prior to closure can also help determine whether ideal vertical placement of the implant has been achieved; if placed too shallow or deep, the implant position can be adjusted.

Hard Tissue Complications

Complications of recipient site in autogenous bone grafting

Autogenous bone grafting of atrophic alveolar ridges in preparation for implant reconstruction is a standard of care in oral and maxillofacial surgery. There are multiple donor sites, including iliac crest, calvarium, rib, tibia, as well as intraoral sites (eg, mandibular symphysis, mandibular ramus, and maxillary tuberosity). Techniques of harvest and complications specific to harvest are beyond the scope of this article. However, complications of the recipient site will be discussed.

Recipient site complications can be broken down into 4 areas:

- Graft contamination
- Wound dehiscence
- Infection
- Resorption

Graft contamination is usually associated with poor handling after harvest. Maintaining principles of sterility is integral to successful graft placement. Once the graft is harvested, avoid using gloves to manipulate the graft; rather transport graft via a

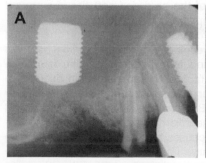
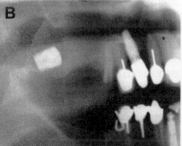
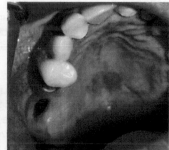

Fig. 2. (*A*) Displacement of implant at time of placement into right maxillary sinus. (*B*) Radiographic presentation at time of retrieval via Caldwell–Luc approach. (*C*) Caldwell Luc approach used for retrieval resulting in Oro-antral fistula requiring second procedure to correct.

secure clamp or forcep from the donor site to a sterile normal saline-filled container. Utilization of sterile water or other transport medium fluids can cause osmotic cell lysis of the graft.[3] If the graft become contaminated, it is best to discard and reharvest.

Wound dehiscence is tantamount to graft failure due to saliva contamination. Incision line dehiscence usually occurs as a result of lack of a tension-free closure or sharp edges of the graft perforating the overlying soft tissue. Considerations prior to grafting include evaluating the soft tissue envelope of recipient area, specifically considering the quality and amount of keratinized mucosa, tissue thickness, and presence of scar tissue. It is important to remember that bone grafting increases volume of underlying bone in the grafted site; evaluating the soft tissue prior to grafting is essential to ensure that the recipient site soft tissue can accommodate the bone graft in a tension-free fashion. In situations where it is suspected that the soft tissue quantity or quality may be questionable, soft tissue grafting or tissue expansion procedures may be indicated. This may provide better quality keratinized tissue in the recipient site (palatal grafts are ideal to increase keratinized tissue). Other issues associated with wound dehiscence include incision design. Ideally, most incisions should be placed on the crest of the alveolar ridge, as this allows for maximal blood supply to the flap. Flaps placed too buccal, palatal, or lingual may have decreased vascular supply, risking necrosis of the flap.[4] Another issue to consider is that by extending existing tissue to cover graft sites, there may be resulting obliteration of the associated vestibule; as such, patients should be made aware of need for a secondary vestibuloplasty as needed. Smoking or existing prosthesis irritation can also be associated with incision dehiscence.

When a dehiscence occurs, treatment options are often based on degree of dehiscence. Small pin-point dehiscences can often be easily managed by local wound care (warm salt water rinses and good hygiene). Larger dehiscences may require nonalcohol-based rinses (alcohol-based rinses can be toxic to nonvascularized bone grafts), local wound care, oral antibiotics to minimize infection risk, and/or debulking of the graft to allow for primary closure. Necrotic graft material should be debrided (**Fig. 3**).

Infections of bone grafts are often associated with poor sterile technique. Prevention of infection is paramount for success of the graft. Appropriate antibiotic coverage intraoperatively and postoperatively is indicated, as is good hygiene and judicious use of alcohol-free oral rinses.

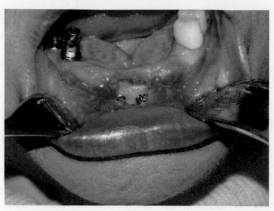

Fig. 3. Dehiscence of soft tissue over graft resulting in graft exposure to oral cavity and subsequent failure. (*Courtesy of* Dr Hani Braidy, Newark, NJ.)

Resorption of bone grafts is common and often has to do with lack of revascularization, often secondary to salivary contamination from wound dehiscence. Cortical bone typically acts as an osteoconductive scaffold for new bone formation. Cancellous bone cells produce bone osteoid, or new bone. The cancellous portion of grafts revascularize much more rapidly than cortical bone.[5] Further, more porous cortical grafts are found to resorb more when compared with denser cortical grafts. Preparing the recipient bed is important to facilitate revascularization. Perforation of the graft site releases growth factors and improves revascularization of the graft. Block grafts require rigid fixation for revascularization. Micromovement can lead to poor revascularization. Fixation can usually be accomplished using a lag screw technique with small titanium screws. When there is resorption of a bone, graft options are limited to trying to use a smaller implant versus regrafting (**Fig. 4**).

Peri-implantitis

"Peri-implantitis is a inflammatory process causing destruction of the hard and soft tissue surround the dental implant."[6] This results in loss of soft tissue and hard tissue support around the dental implant. The etiology is associated with a bacterial biofilm coating the implant. This film has been shown to attach and colonize within minutes to an hour after placement and then exponentially proliferate.[7] Bacteria are usually part of the normal oral flora. The inflammatory response to this biofilm is what causes the bone loss and soft tissue loss. Clinically, implants associated with peri-implantitis can be clinically stable with only radiographic evidence of bone loss, or symptomatic: mobility of implant, purulent or sero-sanguinous

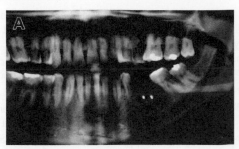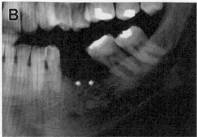

Fig. 4. (*A*) Immediate postoperative panoramic radiograph of symphyseal graft harvested to reconstruct buccal defect in tooth #19/20 site. (*B*) Resorption of graft; sharp edge or superior aspect of graft resulting in wound dehiscence and subsequent resorption of graft.

drainage, foul odor, gingival bleeding, or rarely, pain. In addition, surrounding tissues may appear edematous or tender on examination. On radiographs, there is loss of alveolar bone height; the degree will indicate presence or absence of mobility to the implant.

Prevention of peri-implantitis is primarily on the patient's shoulders to maintain excellent oral hygiene. The surgeon, however, needs to educate the patient on hygiene importance and procedure; further the surgeon and patient must work in concert with the general dentist/dental hygienist in maintaining placed implants and preventing peri-implantitis. Furthermore, once the endosseous implants have been restored, it is the responsibility of the restorative dentist to ensure that the dental prosthesis is easily cleansable and does not create areas for plaque build-up around the implants.

Endosseous implants developing peri-implantitis (clinical suppuration or bone loss radiographically) that are still immobile should be attended to quickly to prevent their failure. Strategies often are based on the degree of bone loss or probing depth. Minimal bone loss and probing depths of less than 4 mm usually require plaque and calculus removal, polishing of the implant crown, and increased oral hygiene visits annually. Mild bone loss and probing depths of 4 to 6 mm require, in addition to increased hygiene visits, chlorhexidine rinses daily or the application of chlorhexidine gels to the affected area. Applying citric acid directly to the exposed implant threads can be considered to detoxify the area. Typically, daily rinsing should be continued until improvement (decreased probing depths) is noted. If probing depths increase beyond 6 mm of significant bone loss (implant still stable), then in addition to hygiene and rinsing, systemic antibiotics focused on gram-negative coverage (metronidazole) is administered for 10 days. Once the any suppuration, edema, and/or infection has resolved, it is reasonable to consider guided tissue regenerative procedures with allogenic bone grafting to restore bone height around the implant.[8] If the implant is restored, the restoration should be taken out of occlusion to minimize functional loads. Mobility of implants results in implant failure, and removal is required with possible bone grafting if desired (**Fig. 5**).

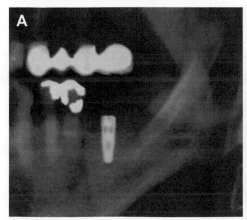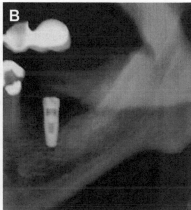

Fig. 5. (*A*) Panoramic radiograph at time of placement of implant. (*B*) Three months after placement greater than 50% bone loss.

REFERENCES

1. Hassani AA, Aighamdi AS. Inferior alveolar nerve injury in implant dentistry: diagnosis, causes, prevention, and management. J Oral Implantol 2010;36:401–7.

2. Misch C, Resnick R. Mandibular neurosensory impairment following dental implant surgery. Management and protocol. Oral Health J 2012;12:1–12.

3. Steiner M, Ramp WK. Short term storage of freshly harvested bone. J Oral Maxillofac Surg 1988;46:868–71.

4. Whetzel TP, Sanders CJ. Arterial anatomy of the oral cavity: an analysis of vascular territories. Plast Reconstr Surg 1997;100:582–7.

5. Manson PN. Facial bone healing and bone grafts. A review of clinical physiology. Clin Plast Surg 1994; 21:331–48.

6. Mombelli A. Microbiology and antimicrobial therapy of peri-implantitis. Periodontol 2000 2002;28: 177–89.

7. Furst MM, Salvi GE, Lang NP, et al. Bacterial colonization immediately after installation on oral titanium implants. Clin Oral Implants Res 2007;18:501–8.

8. Lang NP, Tonetti MS. Peri-implantitis; etiology, pathogenesis, prevention, and therapy. Chapter 7. In: Froum S, editor. Dental implant complication. Ames (IA): Wiley-Blackwell; 2010. p. 119–31.

Digital Technologies for Dental Implant Treatment Planning and Guided Surgery

Alex M. Greenberg, DDS[a,b,*]

KEYWORDS

- Cone beam CT • Dental implant • Oral and maxillofacial surgery • Dental implant surgery

KEY POINTS

- Oral and maxillofacial surgeons now have extraordinary imaging, software planning, and guide fabrication technologies at their disposal to aid in their case selection, clinical decision making, and surgical procedures for dental implant placement.
- Cone beam CT (CBCT) has opened a new era of office-based diagnostic capability and responsibility.
- Improved clinical experiences and evidence-based superior outcomes can be provided with confidence to patients when CT-guided dental implant surgery is used.

New digital technologies have greatly benefited modern dental treatment. The development of dental CBCT scanners from medical helical CT scanners for use in dental offices has given oral and maxillofacial surgeons and their dental colleagues powerful imaging capabilities and software applications. Dental CBCT now allows the implementation of a software-based treatment plan into clinical use through patient-specific, computer-generated, CT-guided drill templates. From a historical perspective, when CT scans were first used to plan dental implant surgery, the first surgical drill guides were handmade by dentists or laboratory technicians from cold cure or processed acrylic, with radiopaque occlusal markers placed prior to the scan and metal drill sleeves placed after the scan. These early surgical drill guides did not have the integration of the CT data into the surgical plan. Klein and colleagues[1,2] and other investigators developed computer planning methods to use fiducial markers to relate the CT scan data to the prosthetic plan and had dental implant drill guides with the placement of planned trajectories based on a technician adjusting a drill press according to the fiducial markers position in 3-D space from the CT scan. This allowed implant trajectories to be placed into the handmade radiographic guide, converting it into a surgical drill guide. Columbia Scientific developed software known as SimPlant, which made planning these cases possible. After the acquisition of Columbia Scientific by Materialise (Leuven, Belgium), which had a process to use the rapid manufactured output from the software-planned dental implant trajectories into the bone made it possible to initially create bone-borne and later tooth-borne surgical drill guides.[3] The use of fan beam CT for the planning of dental implants and the use of

[a] Oral and Maxillofacial Surgery, Columbia University College of Dental Medicine, 630 W. 168th Street, New York, NY 10032, USA; [b] Private Practice Limited to Oral and Maxillofacial Surgery, 18 East 48th Street, Suite 1702, New York, NY 10017, USA
* Private Practice Limited to Oral and Maxillofacial Surgery, 18 East 48th Street, Suite 1702, New York, NY 10017.
E-mail address: nycimplant@aol.com

Oral Maxillofacial Surg Clin N Am 27 (2015) 319–340
http://dx.doi.org/10.1016/j.coms.2015.01.010
1042-3699/15/$ – see front matter © 2015 Elsevier Inc. All rights reserved.

surgical guides for CT-guided dental implant placement had become possible. Use of the dual-scan process was first described for the completely edentulous by Jacobs and colleagues[4] and Van Steenberghe and colleagues,[5] who first recognized the potential for CT rapid prototyped surgical guides for complete denture patients.[6,7] After the CT scan of a patient with a barium-impregnated radiographic guide, bone-borne surgical drill guides were fabricated to fit stereolithographic jaw models that required the opening of a flap for placement of dental implants. Materialise then developed the next generation of surgical drill guides that had bone trajectories merged by surface-to-surface matching with an optical scan of a dental model.[8] The surgical drill guide could then be created by rapid prototyping, which was then tooth-borne. Feldman[9] with iDent Imaging (New York, New York) furthered the development of dual-scan process for the partially edentulous with an artifact-corrected image to create a postsegmentation surgical guide that could be tooth- or mucosal-borne. Instead of using barium, the dual-scan surgical guide process uses the registration of radiodense fiducial radiographic markers, such as metal beads or guttapercha, from the scan of the radiographic guide in a patient's mouth (**Fig. 1**) and from a separate scan of the radiographic guide in a Styrofoam box or stand aligned in the same orientation (**Fig. 2**). These 2 data sets that that can be merged through the registration of the fiducial markers and permits the creation of an artifact-corrected image. The 2 data sets of digitized images are uploaded to the company for file conversion and are merged in the planning software, with registration and superimposition of the radiographic template to the bone images. iDent Imaging, Nobel Biocare (Yorba Linda, California), and other companies developed the first commercial dual-scan tooth-borne surgical drill guides with virtual

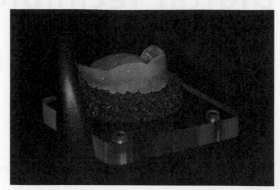

Fig. 2. Radiographic guide on Styrofoam for CBCT scan.

insertion of drill trajectories manufactured by rapid prototyping manufacturing. When using these software programs, it may be necessary to modify the voxel settings of the CBCT so that the data are obtained in the right DICOM format that needs to be used by the planning software. The planning software vendor should be checked carefully to obtain their scanning protocol. These 2 DICOM data sets are then exported from the CBCT scanner by a custom export plug-in and transferred as data files for uploading to the vendor. The data are uploaded to the master site software, or the software may need to be converted by third-party service vendors or the software vendor itself, which may require the payment of a fee for conversion and can include set-up of the case for review by a clinician, who ultimately must make the final approval regarding the case and the production of the surgical drill guide.

Materialise's software SimPlant has a barium-impregnated scan appliance created and scanned as the first data set; then a model is sent to Materialise for optical scanning so that an artifact-free image of the teeth can be created as a second data set. After the merger of the data sets, a surgical drill guide is made according to the planned implant position(s) in the treatment planning software.

There are many treatment planning software programs and providers of surgical guides, with some closed systems associated with particular implant systems, whereas others are open platforms for use with all dental implants. Some software programs, such as Cybermed (Irvine, California) and Blue Sky Bio (Grayslake, Illinois), may not require a radiographic scan appliance and can surface-to-surface merge either from a CBCT scan of a dental model or an optical scan of a patient's dentition for the fabrication of a surgical drill guide. In the case of Blue Sky Bio, this process is via a rapid printed model on which a

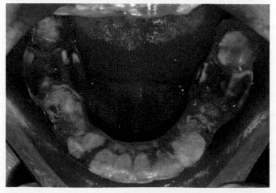

Fig. 1. Radiographic guide in a patient's mouth for CBCT scan. (*Courtesy of* Dr. Mark Hamburger, London, UK.)

vacuum-formed template is created with drill sleeves attached to a trajectory from the model.

It is critically important when using laboratory or dual-scan methods for surgical guides that an accurate dental model is created to ensure that a well-fitting radiographic guide is fabricated (**Fig. 3**). These radiographic guides must fit the dentition and edentulous ridges well so that a correct seating of the radiographic guide is achieved during the CT scan of a patient. For dual-scan protocol, the placement of fiducial radiodense markers in the radiographic guide is necessary to allow the registration or matching of the 2 data sets. Materials, such as iNterra (Dentsply, Tulsa, Oklahoma), have been found to allow the fabrication of a chairside radiographic guide the same day that an CBCT in an office setting is performed (**Fig. 4**). INTERRA is a cost-effective, light-cured composite material that comes in small, medium, and large horseshoe-formed sizes and can be shaped and light cured in the mouth without the need for an impression and creation of a dental cast. The material is molded with finger pressure to obtain the occlusal surfaces of the teeth with adequate coverage for positive seating of the appliance during CBCT scanning and extension for a palatal or lingual flange for the insertion of radiographic markers placed closer to the vestibular depth/inferior border of the guide. As with cold cure or laboratory-processed radiographic guides, radiographic markers are placed distant to teeth so that dental restorations scatter artifact does not obscure them. iNterra is then light cured in the mouth and once the radiographic markers are added, a radiographic guide is created. Denture teeth or other crown forms can be cold cure or light cure bonded to the INTERRA material so that a radiographic guide with teeth appears in the CBCT. INTERRA allows a CBCT to be performed with a radiographic guide in the same visit, with the next visit for CT-guided implant surgery, thus shortening the process.

Essential to treatment planning for dental implants is completely reviewing all the images of the CBCT scan in addition to the sagittal oblique and panoramic images. Depending on the scanner, there often is an initial video sequence scanning through the complete image of a patient slice by slice. Scrolling through this axial plane stack of slices allows an initial overview of patient data to detect any pathologic lesions. Once this initial review is complete, it is possible to review and, if necessary, adjust the spline cut that has been placed through the axial view of the specific jaw, either the maxilla or the mandible, so that an adequate panoramic view is seen. For example, a correct spline cut improves the visualization of the mandibular canal. This panoramic view should then be viewed in an orderly manner, viewing the bony structures, including the bilateral condyles and the outline of the jaw. In the mandible, this includes the mandibular canals in the maxilla sinus, cavities. Tooth decay, periodontal disease, periapical pathology, impacted teeth, and other pathologic lesions should be noted and further evaluated. Once the panoramic image has been viewed, there should be a review of the coronal, axial, and sagittal views to complete the evaluation for the presence of any pathologic lesions or to look for the problem that the scan was intended for. If an internal or external sinus lift is performed, it is important to evaluate the sinus cavities for the presence of mucosal thickening, polyps, mucoceles, air/fluid levels, or septae. The coronal views can also be helpful to relate the arches to each other and positioning for dental implants depending on the surgical plan.

CBCT can be helpful for patients undergoing comprehensive dental implant treatment to develop a basic understanding of their dental disease, including which teeth may need to be removed, periodontal disease to be treated, degree of bone atrophy in edentulous sites (**Fig. 5**A, B), gross decay, position of the mandibular canals

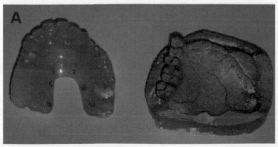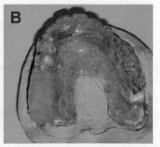

Fig. 3. (*A*, *B*) Examples of well fitting radiographic guide with correct dental anatomy with 6 gutta-percha markers. (*A*) Radiographic guide and dental cast. (*B*) Radiographic guide correctly fitting on dental cast.

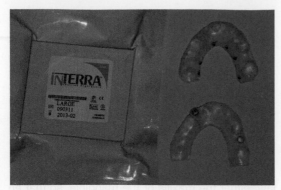

Fig. 4. INTERRA package and radiographic and surgical guides. Right package, upper left radiographic guide, lower left surgical guide.

that can be mapped (see **Fig. 5**C, D), the quality and quantity of subantral bone, and what the residual bone will be in sites where teeth are to be removed for delayed or immediate dental implant placement. Advanced scanning methods involve the use of scan appliances so that the planned prosthetic outcome can be related to the bone sites for immediate and delayed dental implant placement with site development.

When using CBCT to evaluate dental implant patients, there are several methods to view and interpret the images. Most CBCT scanners provide views in the axial, coronal, and sagittal planes with the ability to view in real time images in a 3-panel window to allow a 3-D representation of a patient. This 3-D viewing can be further visualized with 3-D volume rendering, also a feature of most modern CBCT scanners, the extent of which depends on the size of the field of view. The initial viewing window of most CBCT software programs is the panoramic image with a corresponding axial view with an adjustable spline. A spline is a continuous semicircular line within the axial plane that defines the panoramic view by selecting the panoramic image depth of view from buccal to lingual. It is useful in helping to define images, such as the mandibular canals, by selecting the correct sagittal cut through the mandible. A clinician can reset the spline using points moved by the mouse to establish the desired panoramic view through the maxilla or the mandible. Once the panoramic view is set, it is possible to enter a window displaying the panoramic view and the oblique sagittal views of the maxilla or the mandible. The oblique sagittal views of the jaw can be likened to slicing a banana and viewing the cross-sections. The oblique sagittal views allow the visualization of the buccal to lingual or labial to palatal width of bone and whether there is adequate width to place dental implants. Vertical dimension

can be measured and structures, such as the mandibular canal, mental foramen, and anterior canal loop, can be visualized.[10–12] There can be considerable variation in the mental foramen and its position as well as visualization related to bone density, especially in the edentulous and partially edentulous (**Fig. 6**).[13] In the completely edentulous, the mental foramen can be often found at the alveolar crest[14] (**Fig. 7**) and the identification and preservation of this important structure relates to the placement of incisions and soft tissue dissection to avoid nerve injury. Accessory mental foramina have been observed in 7% of patients.[15] Mandibular incisive canals are observed in 93% of CT scans according to 1 study.[16] Bifid mandibular canals have been observed in 15.6% of patients.[17] Canal estimation is generally manually performed and software performs an estimation based on selected endpoints and when completed fills the canal with color, which is helpful for visualization to both clinician and patient. Maxillary regional structures, such as the sinuses,[18] pterygoid plate,[19] nasal floor, and incisive foramen[20] (**Fig. 8**), are other key aspects to be visualized. Sinus disease may be represented by thickened lining mucosa, periapical lesions, mucoceles, antroliths, inspissated mucous, impacted teeth with or without cysts, and air/fluid levels of infection. Periodontal infections can also be associated with oroantral communications, which can be further evaluated in the axial and coronal views. The incisive foramen often has variability in width ranging from 1.8 to 5.5 mm.[20] This variation in incisive foramen size and location can influence the ability to place dental implants at the maxillary central incisor sites. Widened incisive foramina on posteroanterior radiographs are often mistakenly identified as nasopalatine cysts, which are uncommon lesions and well visualized by CBCT. Considerable variation is often present in the maxillary sinus anatomy, which, for example, in the sinus, may be limited to the molar region and in some patients can extend as far forward as the canines. The presence of antral floor septae also has clinical importance because it relates to the ability to perform sinus lift surgery.[21–23]

Many CBCT machines have software that allows the manual placement of dental implant images in the panoramic and oblique sagittal views, without correlation to surgical guide appliances. As discussed previously, when viewing images of interest for dental implant planning, it is of critical importance to evaluate all the windows to ensure that no pathologic entities or lesions are missed. This is important not only for the correct treatment of patients but also for medicolegal reasons. A

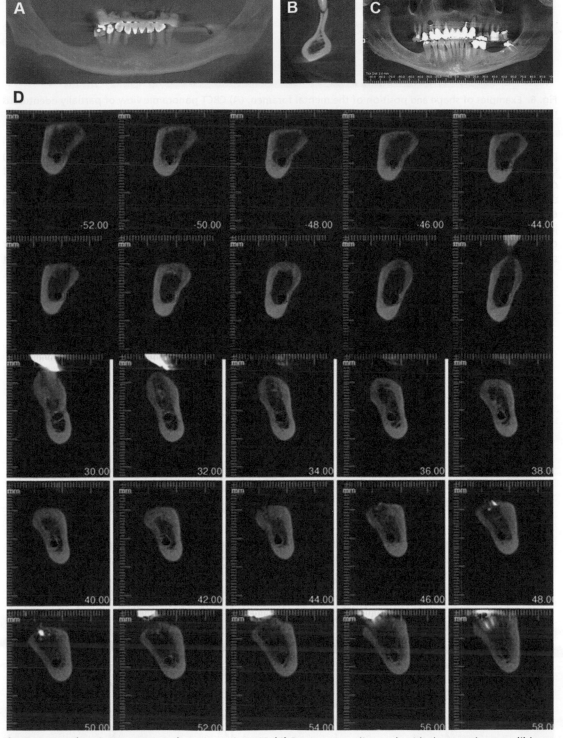

Fig. 5. Comprehensive treatment planning with CBCT. (*A*) Panoramic radiograph with the anterior mandible appearing to have a large amount of vertical bone height. (*B*) Sequential oblique sagittal cross-sectional image of anterior mandible with significantly reduced buccal-lingual bone width. (*C*) Panoramic view of the bilateral posterior mandibular edentulous ridges with bilateral mandibular canal mapping in gray. (*D*) Sequential oblique sagittal cross-sectional images with mandibular canal mapped.

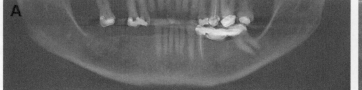
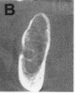

Fig. 6. Examples of shape and position of the mental foramen. (*A*) CBCT panoramic view of partially edentulous mandible in class III bone. (*B*) CBCT sequential oblique cross-sectional view of the mental foramen in class III bone.

practitioner can also have an outside medical or dental radiologist review the CBCT to ensure thorough review of the images. Other dental problems, such as endodontic lesions, caries, periodontal disease, impacted teeth, and temporomandibular joint findings, need to be noted. Hounsfield units can be helpful in determining the bone density and in the range of type I highly cortical bone to type IV highly osteopenic bone is present,[23] which can be observed even within the different levels of the vertical and horizontal dimensions of the alveolar process.[24] Bone density can also affect the ability to visualize structures, such as the mandibular canal, which diminishes with decreased bone density. Teeth that may appear on panoramic or posteroanterior views to have bone attachment

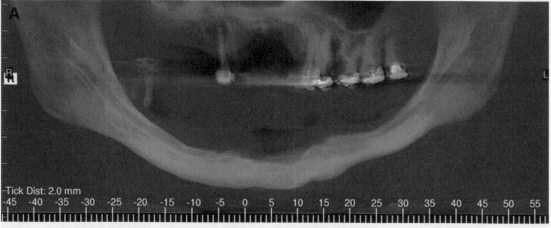

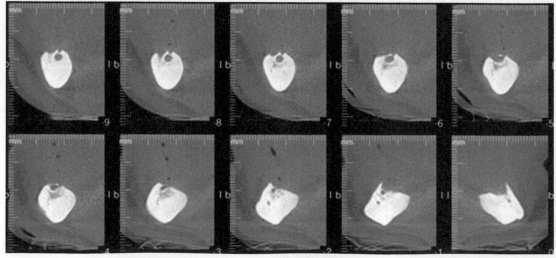

Fig. 7. (*A*) Panoramic view of totally edentulous mandible, class I bone. (*B*) Sequential oblique sagittal cross-sectional images of edentulous mandible, class I bone with mental foramen at crest of ridge.

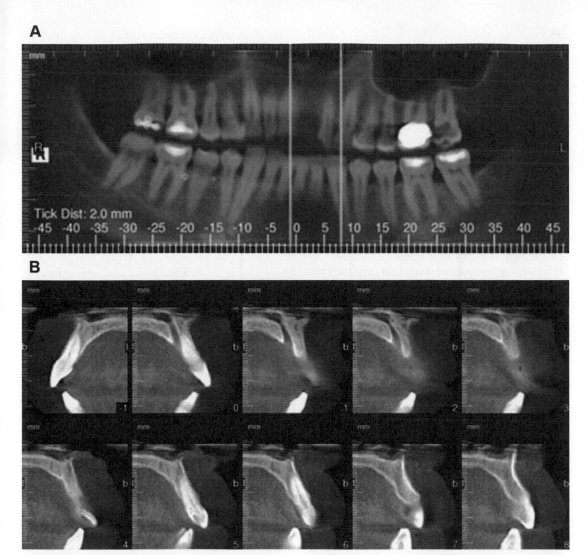

Fig. 8. CBCT views of the incisive foramen. (*A*) Panoramic view parallel blue lines delineate the region for sequential oblique sagittal cross sectional images. (*B*) Sequential oblique sagittal cross sectional images.

can be found as floating teeth without any bone attachment that can only be visualized by CBCT. In such cases of advanced ridge resorption, there may or may not be a requirement for bone grafting of defects, depending on the residual alveolar ridge dimensions. General needs for bone grafting can be coordinated with dental implant treatment planning and CT-guided surgery because there are many patients for whom these procedures are performed in stages with the essential need for comprehensive treatment planning, including the planned removal of teeth, temporary provisionalization, mini-implants, complex bone grafting, and staged dental implant placement.

Inferior alveolar nerve injuries are a potential complication and a known risk in posterior mandibular dental implant placement. In cases of

an injured inferior alveolar nerve and terminated procedure because of patient complaint or operator concern, on a postoperative CBCT it can be observed in the oblique sagittal reconstruction as the loss of canal anatomy, usually at the superior aspect of the canal because of overpenetration of the drill bit. For example, in this patients the dental implants were placed too deeply into the mandible with impingement on the mandibular canal along its superior, medial, or lateral aspects can be observed (**Fig. 9** A). In either of these situations, canal estimation with color can be helpful in documenting these problems. The avoidance of penetration of the mandibular canal (see **Fig. 9**B) and inferior alveolar nerve injuries is one of the most important indications for CBCT imaging of the posterior mandible and CT-guided dental

A

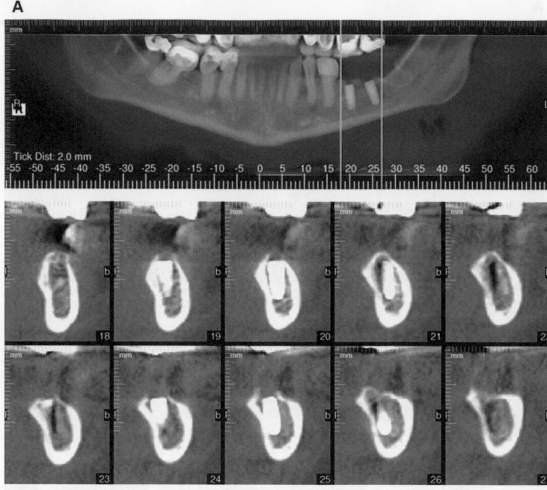

Fig. 9. (*A*) CBCT Panoramic view of dental implants placed too deep into the left mandible with impingement on mandibular canal. Parallel blue lines delineate the region for sequential oblique sagittal cross sectional images. (*B*) Sequential oblique sagittal cross sectional images of dental implant overpenetration of drill bit without implant placement with superior aspect of mandibular canal removed. (*C*) CBCT Panoramic view of right posterior mandible with overpenetration of drill bit into the mandibular canal without placement of dental implants.

implant surgery, which can allow drill depth control.

The advantage of surgical guidance planning systems is that they allow the integration of CT data with the surgical procedure, which is carried out through the use of the surgical drill guide. Initially, handmade surgical drill guides were at best estimations based solely on tooth position without the benefit of integrated CT scan imaging concerning the exact bone anatomy. Handmade surgical drill guides allowed surgeons with the image of the bone in their mind's eye to have improved implant positions based on the prosthetic plan. Through sophisticated software, CT guidance allows the complete integration of dental implant drilling with correct trajectories that have

been preplanned to the exact bony anatomy. Depending on the dental implant system instrumentation, drilling depth can be controlled as well (**Fig. 10**). These systems use a drill guide handle that fits into a master sleeve and allows for the changes of the diameter of the drill bit in the series of drills used to create the osteotomy. These systems also allow the placement of dental implants through the drill guide master sleeves so that the entire procedure can be performed flapless. By using a tissue punch that cores out the gingiva overlying the planned osteotomy site, flapless surgery allows dental implants to be placed, thus reducing operating time and postoperative pain and swelling. It is also possible through a retrofit of the surgical drill guide to place a

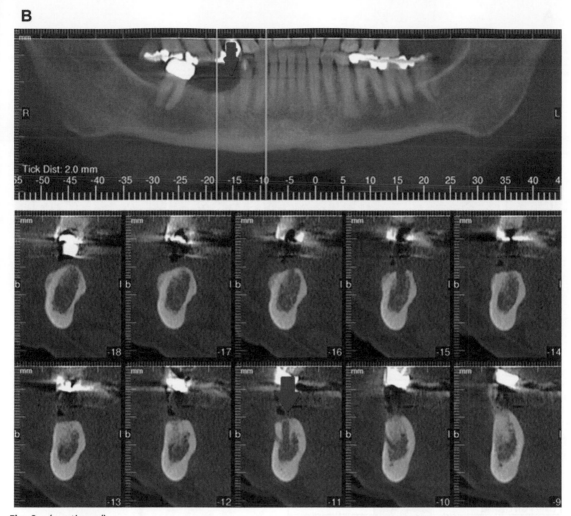

Fig. 9. (*continued*)

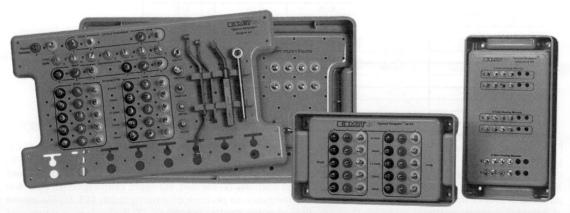

Fig. 10. Navigator CT-guided dental implant surgery instrument tray. (*Courtesy of* Biomet 3i, West Palm Beach, FL; with permission.)

A

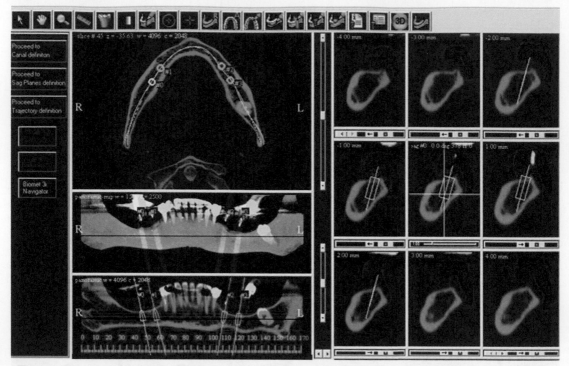

B

Patient Name	
Id	327890
Gender	F
D.O.B	
Clinical ref#	
Date printed	
Date of scan	
Date Plan created	
Dentist name	
Notes	

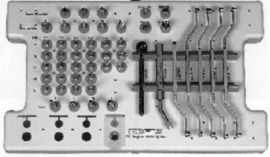

Implant Label	0	1	2	3
Implant Code	IOSS485	IOSS485	IOSS485	IOSS485
Implant Length (mm)	8.50	8.50	8.50	8.50
Implant Diameter (mm)	4.00	4.00	4.00	4.00
Depth Line	12.00	12.00	12.00	12.00
Tissue Punch	4.00	4.00	4.00	4.00
Countersink	4.00	4.00	4.00	4.00
Drill / Handle One	2.00B/4A	2.00B/4A	2.00B/4A	2.00B/4A
Drill / Handle Two	3.25B/4B	3.25B/4B	3.25B/4B	3.25B/4B
Drill / Handle Three	N/A	N/A	N/A	N/A
Tap	4.00	4.00	4.00	4.00
Implant Mount	4.00/12.00	4.00/12.00	4.00/12.00	4.00/12.00
Bone Profiler	4.00	4.00	4.00	4.00
Analog Mount	4.00/12.00	4.00/12.00	4.00/12.00	4.00/12.00

Fig. 11. Case report of bilateral posterior mandibular edentulous ridge dental implant placement via flapless CT-guided surgery. (*A*) Software window with registered radiographic guide to mandible bone window with planned dental implant trajectories teeth #18, #19, #30, and #31. (*B*) Software report detailing Navigator (Biomet 3i, West Palm Beach, Florida) instrumentation specific for each dental implant. (*C*) Rapid prototyped surgical drill guide with master sleeves. (*D*) Use of drill handle and handpiece to perform osteotomy tooth #18. (*E*) Placement of 4 dental implants posterior mandible through surgical guide flapless procedure. (*F*) Postoperative panoramic radiograph demonstrates excellent parallelism of dental implants placed superior to the bilateral mandibular canals. ([*A, B*] *Courtesy of* iDent Imaging, New York, NY.)

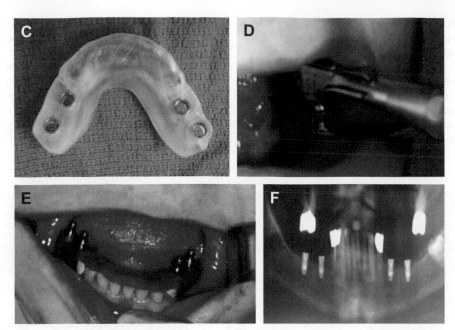

Fig. 11. (*continued*)

prefabricated temporary dental prosthesis.[6,25] Single anterior teeth can have superior aesthetics with the immediate placement of provisional restoration.[26,27] The All-on-4 method, as described by Maló and colleagues,[28] provides for the immediate provisionalization of the full arch in the completely edentulous. Other investigators have also described immediate loading of full-arch temporary prostheses as well as final prostheses.[29,30] Increased failure rates with immediate provisional loading of dental implants has been reported.[31] This author has also found, in a small unpublished pilot series using CT-guided 2-stage implant surgery, that success rate is also improved with fewer failures because the osteotomy sites are more perfectly circular as opposed to ovoid forms obtained by freehand drilling, which improves implant thread engagement, and dental implants are placed more reliably within the center of the bone. Precise osteotomies are less traumatic to the bone, which may also contribute to improved success rate of implants placed with surgical guides. By preserving vascular supply, flapless surgery may improve the maintenance of crestal bone when using the biomechanical and biological width advantages of internal connected dental implants.

A major advantage of CT-guided dental implant surgery is the precise knowledge of the underlying important anatomic structures. For example, in the mandible this relates to the position of the mandibular canals and the ability during dental

implant placement to avoid injury to the mandibular canal and mental foramen.[32] This avoidance of mandibular nerve injury is achievable by using customized dental implant instrument systems for use with the surgical drill guide that allow depth control with drill stops on the drills at specific lengths and precise placement of dental implants, with specialized fixture mounts with the prolongation based on known variations in gingival thickness (**Fig. 11**). In the maxilla, sinus

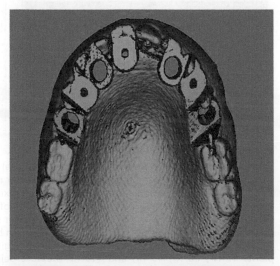

Fig. 12. Example of screw fixation trajectories in a surgical guide.

perforation and avoidance of the incisive canal can be prevented through foreknowledge of the CBCT scan images and use of surgical drill guides.

Fixation of surgical guides with screws or pins is also an important consideration. A well-fitting guide may be held in the mouth by an operator while drilling takes place, which requires holding both the drill handle and the surgical drill guide with the nondominant hand, which can also be performed by an assistant, and drilling with the dominant hand. Fixation of the guide with pins or screws can be incorporated in many guide systems as preplanned trajectories (**Fig. 12**), allowing clinicians freedom to use both hands without having to hold down the surgical drill guide, and ensures a more precise fit. When multiple implants are placed, insertion of the first 2 dental implants through the

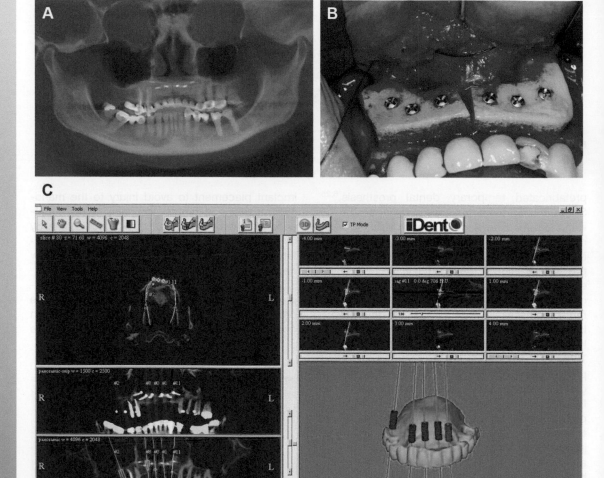

Fig. 13. (*A–J*) Case report demonstrating use of surgical guide in a bone-grafted deficient anterior partially edentulous maxillary ridge. (*A*) Panoramic view of anterior maxillary defect reconstructed with iliac crest bone graft. (*B*) Clinical of iliac crest onlay bone grafts anterior maxillary defect. (*C*) Software planning with virtual guide and planned implant trajectories after 6 months' healing of bone grafts. The guide will be digitally converted into a drill guide for rapid printing of an STL file and master sleeve insertion. (*D*) Radiographic guide. (*E*) Surgical drill guide. (*F*) Surgical procedure with surgical guide try-in before removal of fixations screws. Note satisfactory healing of block bone grafts. (*G*) Intraoperative use of surgical drill guide. (*H*) Intraoperative placement of dental implants #7 NP, #8 RP, #9 RP, and #10 RP (Replace Select, Nobel Biocare, Yorba Linda, CA). (*I*) Postoperative panoramic radiograph reveals excellent parallelism of implants. (*J*) Final implant supported maxillary prosthesis. ([*C*] *Courtesy of* iDent Imaging, New York, NY.)

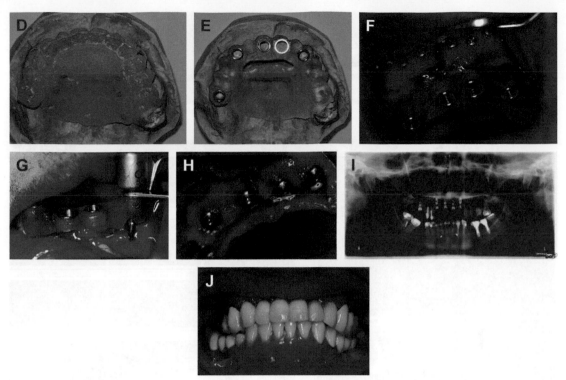

Fig. 13. (*continued*)

master sleeves can also be a method for securing the surgical drill guide.

Clinicians find that as a result of using CT guidance there is a great improvement in dental implant positions, seen as better parallelism between implants (**Fig. 13**A–J), improved implant position relative to crown or bridge prosthetic anatomy, less impingement on periodontal structures of adjacent teeth, and less reliance of what can be mistaken to appear by direct vision as the best path of implant insertion relative to the adjacent teeth. Many experienced clinicians believe that they can place dental implants perfectly without the use of surgical drill guides, which usually require a flap. On critical review, however, of nonguided dental implant placement using postoperative radiographs and the observation later on at stage II uncovering with abutment placement, many of these implants could have been placed in better positions.[33] CT guidance allows much greater accuracy in implant placement because of the presurgical planning experience, which is transferred into the surgical guide drill template with the avoidance of freehand imprecision, especially in aesthetic cases (**Fig. 14**A–L).

There are disadvantages to the use of CT guidance, including the technical learning curve, use of the software, digital or traditional impression taking, and the additional cost of both a radiographic guide and a surgical guide. Learning to trust the surgical plan and the guide also can be considered an initial disadvantage. Many clinicians today own and operate a CBCT, which is also part of the technical learning curve that relates to gaining improved knowledge of CT scanning. It also takes time to learn how to operate a CT scanner and maintain its calibration, understand how to convert files and export data, and prepare files for uploading into the software.[34] Reading a CBCT requires continuing education as well as time and experience to understand what is looked at and looked for. Reading can be aided by sending these studies to either a dental or medical radiologist for a report to share the medicolegal responsibility, especially if scans are performed for other practitioners. Using dental implant planning software can add cost as well as the time and experience necessary to learn the technical aspects of these programs and their subtleties. Design of the case improves as experience is gained and through collaboration with restorative dentists. Online interactive meetings between clinicians is highly recommended, which are helpful in obtaining understanding of both parties as to the treatment plan that is desired. Collaboration with dental

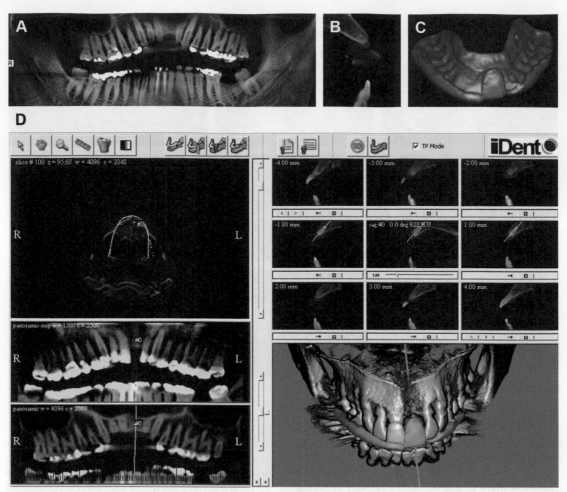

Fig. 14. (A–L) Single-tooth aesthetic zone case report. (A) Preoperative panoramic radiograph of missing tooth #9. (B) Preoperative sequential oblique cross-sectional image of anterior maxilla edentulous ridge tooth #9. (C) Radiographic template. (D) Software planning with virtual radiographic guide and planned dental implant trajectory with 3-D bone window. (E) Software planning with virtual radiographic guide and planned dental implant trajectory. (F) Software planning with virtual surgical drill guide and planned dental implant trajectory. (G) Surgical drill guide. (H) Intraoperative use of surgical drill guide. (I) Intraoperative placement of dental implant. (J) Postoperative placement of healing abutment with satisfactory soft tissue aesthetics. (K) Postoperative periapical radiograph with satisfactory osseointegration of dental implant and crown tooth #9. (L) Clinical view of final crown tooth #9 with satisfactory aesthetics. ([D–F, H] Courtesy of iDent Imaging, New York, NY.)

laboratory technicians and consultation with more experienced colleagues may also be useful in the planning of more complicated cases.

The need for CT guidance is well understood; Almog and colleagues[35,36] in their study found a difference between the planned prosthetic trajectory and the residual bone trajectory, which is the disparity between what seemed to be the ideal bone thickness and the bone thickness dictated by the correct prosthetic trajectory for the dental implant. This finding supports the importance of the use of CT guidance for dental implant

placement. An example of less ideal implant placement is a case of hybrid fixed dental implant prosthetics, in which implants are placed too labial and the retention screws can only be placed through the labial aspect, resulting in a maintenance and aesthetic problem. The lack of parallelism or space between implants can also result in compromised prosthetic results and hygiene issues.

CT guidance can be critical for the correct implant placement in immediate extraction implant cases. The planning for immediate extraction and

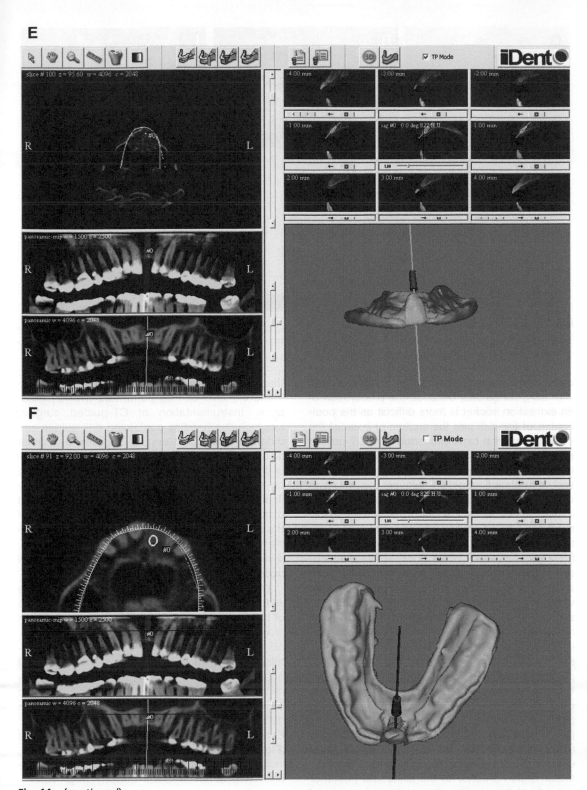

Fig. 14. (*continued*)

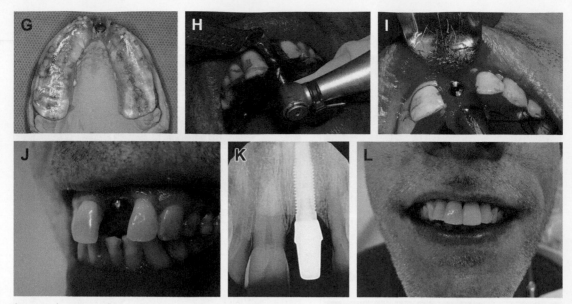

Fig. 14. (*continued*)

dental implant placement can be better idealized with surgical guides, because the preparation of an extraction socket is more difficult as the positioning of the drill into the septum or base of the socket can be a blind procedure.[37] If CT-guided surgical planning is used, there is foreknowledge of the amount of bone apical to the socket for secure implant fixation. CT software planning provides the precise location in the socket where the implant should be placed for prosthetic guidance, need for bone grafting, and possible immediate temporization. Maxillary double-rooted premolars have greater width in the buccal-palatal dimensions with thin inter-radicular septae that require an implant to be placed in the palatal root socket, which may be less ideal if it is not centered in the socket, which is most ideal for crown placement. In cases of immediate extraction of a molar and implant to be placed, determination of adequate septal bone and the ideal trajectory can be better planned and actualized by CT guidance.

Using dental implant planning software it is possible to plan sinus lift bone grafting[38] and dental implant placement. It is also possible to place dental implants at angulations that preclude the need for sinus lift bone grafting by using available bone, if it is adequate, in the premolar region anterior to the sinus and posterior aspects of the maxillary tuberosity and pterygoid plate. Often these implants are placed at greater angulations, which can be compensated for by the use of custom abutments.[39] These abutment angles can also be planned in coordination with

the prosthetic design. The placement of zygomatic implants can be performed with CT guidance. Instrumentation of CT-guided surgical kits includes handles containing drill guides and different drill diameters for the use of master sleeves. Master sleeves also allow the insertion of the dental implants on fixture mounts based on a prolongation formula that accounts for the final depth of the dental implant, thickness of overlying gingiva, and height of the sleeve of the surgical guide. For the fully edentulous, overdenture cases with ball attachments, clip bars, mini-implants, or combinations of these are all possible with CT guidance.

The use of dental implant planning software with CT guidance is extremely helpful in cases of bone grafting necessary to augment a deficient alveolar ridge prior to the placement of dental implants. The software allows clinicians to determine how much bone is present in quality and quantity, whether bone graft augmentation is necessary, and, if so, how much bone needs to be grafted to place dental implants in specific deficient sites and at the correct trajectories. Examples include class III ridge relationships (**Fig. 15**A–M) in which a fixed case is desired, individual cases of buccal plate loss with severe buccolingual/buccopalatal atrophy (**Fig. 16**A–F), lack of vertical bone height, and subantral bone deficiency.

Oral and maxillofacial surgeons now have extraordinary imaging, software planning, and guide fabrication technologies at their disposal to

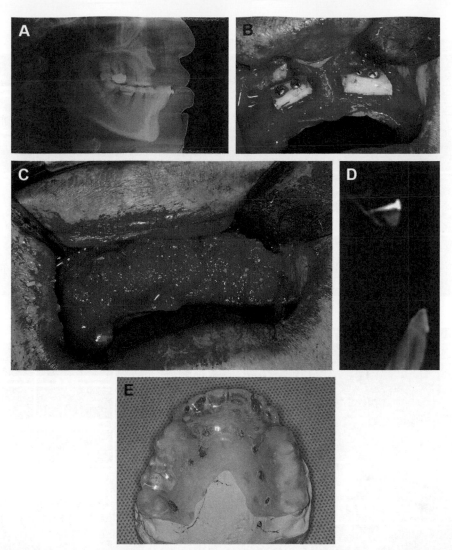

Fig. 15. (*A–F*) Case report demonstrating use of surgical guide in a bone-grafted deficient anterior partially edentulous maxillary ridge. (*A*) Lateral cephalometric radiograph demonstrates clinical class III ridge relationship. (*B*) Bilateral mandibular ramus cortical bone grafts with screw fixation for augmentation of anterior maxillary ridge. (*C*) Autogenous mandibular scraped bone graft covering the bilateral mandibular ramus cortical bone grafts, which was then covered with resorbable collagen membrane. (*D*) Postoperative sagittal view of CBCT that reveals adequate bone graft healing and satisfactory augmentation of ridge. (*E*) Radiographic guide with planned prosthetic tooth setup. (*F*) Planning software using postoperative CT scan demonstrating panoramic view of dental implant planned trajectories Radiographic guide. (*G*) Planning software using postoperative CT scan demonstrating panoramic view of dental implant planned trajectories with virtual creation of surgical drill guide. (*H*) Surgical template. (*I*) Try-in of surgical template in the mouth. (*J*) Intraoperative exposure of mandibular ramus block bone grafts with satisfactory healing. (*K*) Surgical procedure with surgical guide. (*L*) Intraoperative placement of dental implants #6, #7, #8, #9, #10, and #11, with precise positions achieved. (*M*) Postoperative periapical radiograph reveals excellent parallelism of dental implants teeth #6, #7, and #8. (*N*) Postoperative periapical radiograph reveals excellent parallelism of dental implants teeth #9, #10, and #11. (*Courtesy of [F, G]* iDent Imaging, New York, NY.)

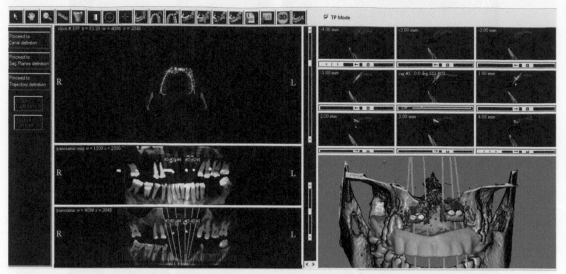

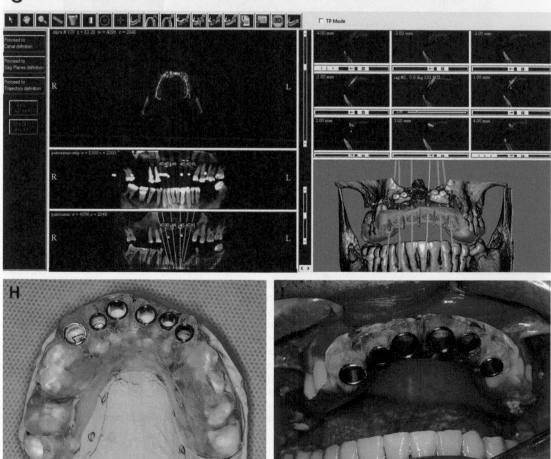

Fig. 15. (*continued*)

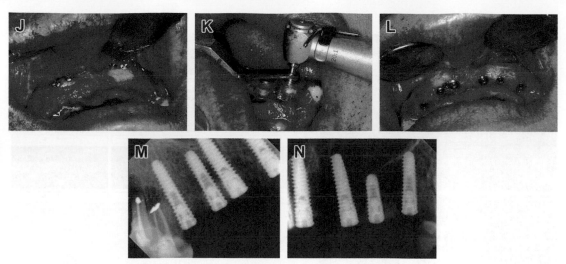

Fig. 15. (*continued*)

aid in case selection, clinical decision making, and surgical procedures for dental implant placement. CBCT has opened a new era of office-based diagnostic capability and responsibility. Improved clinical experiences and evidence-based superior outcomes can be provided with confidence to patients when CT-guided dental implant surgery is used.[40]

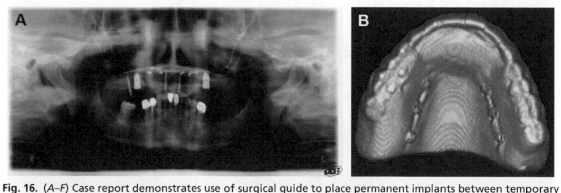

Fig. 16. (*A–F*) Case report demonstrates use of surgical guide to place permanent implants between temporary mini-implants and other previously placed permanent implants in a bone-grafted case with inadequate buccal-palatal dimensions. (*A*) Panoramic view of initially placed dental implants #5 and #12 with mini-implants #4, #8, and #9 for overdenture retention. (*B*) Maxillary complete denture as radiographic template with 6 fiducial markers added. (*C*) Software planning with virtual radiographic guide of denture with planned trajectories. (*D*) Software window with registered radiographic guide to mandible bone window with planned dental implant trajectories teeth #6, #7, #10, and #11. (*E*) Close-up view of software planning with virtual radiographic guide of denture with planned trajectories. (*F*) Surgical guide. (*G*) Incisions and positioning of surgical guide prior to bone graft fixation screw removal. (*H*) Intraoperative use of iTool handled drill guide instrument with surgical guide. (*I*) Placement of dental implants with precise positions. (*J*) Postoperative panoramic radiograph demonstrates parallelism of dental implants teeth #5, #6, #11, and #12 and avoidance of impingement on mini-implants #4, #8, and #9 and permanent implants #4 and #13. (*K*) Postoperative clinical stage II healing abutment placement occlusal view reveals satisfactory implant spacing. ([*C–E*] *Courtesy of* iDent Imaging, New York, NY.)

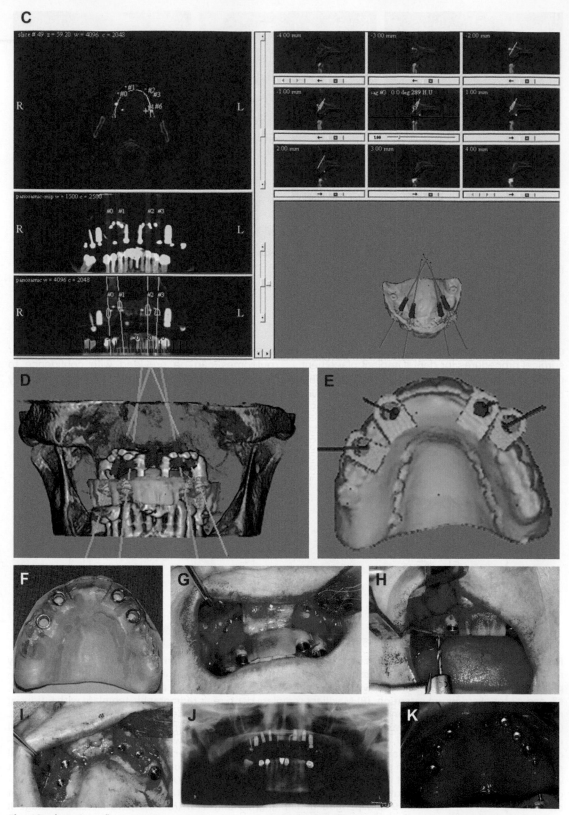

Fig. 16. (*continued*)

REFERENCES

1. Klein M, Abrams M. Computer-guided surgery utilizing a computer-milled surgical template. Pract Proced Aesthet Dent 2001;13(2):165–9.

2. Klein M, Cranin AN, Sirakian A. A computerized tomography (CT) scan appliance for optimal presurgical and preprosthetic planning of the implant patient. Pract Periodontics Aesthet Dent 1993;5(6):33–9.

3. Tardieu PB, Vrielinck L, Escolano E, et al. Computer-assisted implant placement: scan template, simplant, surgiguide, and SAFE system. Int J Periodontics Restorative Dent 2007;27(2):141–9.

4. Jacobs R, Adriansens A, Naert I, et al. Predictability of reformatted computed tomography for preoperative planning of endosseous implants. Dentomaxillofac Radiol 1999;28(1):37–41.

5. van Steenberghe D, Naert I, Andersson M, et al. A custom template and definitive prosthesis allowing immediate implant loading in the maxilla: a clinical report. Int J Oral Maxillofac Implants 2002;17(5):663–70.

6. van Steenberghe D, Glauser R, Blombäck U, et al. A computed tomographic scan-derived customized surgical template and fixed prosthesis for flapless surgery and immediate loading of implants in fully edentulous maxillae: a prospective multicenter study. Clin Implant Dent Relat Res 2005;7(Suppl 1):S111–20.

7. Verstreken K, Van Cleynenbreugel J, Martens K, et al. An image-guided planning system for endosseous oral implants. IEEE Trans Med Imaging 1998;17(5):842–52.

8. Rosenfeld AL, Mandelaris GA, Tardieu PB. Prosthetically directed implant placement using computer software to ensure precise placement and predictable prosthetic outcomes. Part 1: diagnostics, imaging, and collaborative accountability. Int J Periodontics Restorative Dent 2006;26(3):215–21.

9. US Patent 7,574,025.

10. Uchida Y, Noguchi N, Goto M, et al. Measurement of anterior loop length for the mandibular canal and diameter of the mandibular incisive canal to avoid nerve damage when installing endosseous implants in the interforaminal region: a second attempt introducing cone beam computed tomography. J Oral Maxillofac Surg 2009;67(4):744–50.

11. Froum S, Casanova L, Byrne S, et al. Risk assessment prior to extraction for immediate implant placement in the posterior mandible - a computerized tomographic scan study. J Periodontol 2010;82(3):395–402.

12. De Andrade E, Otomo-Corgel J, Pucher J, et al. The intraosseous course of the mandibular incisive nerve in the mandibular symphysis. Int J Periodontics Restorative Dent 2001;21(6):591–7.

13. Bou Serhal C, Jacobs R, Flygare L, et al. Perioperative validation of localisation of the mental foramen. Dentomaxillofac Radiol 2002;31(1):39–43.

14. Soikkonen K, Wolf J, Ainamo A, et al. Changes in the position of the mental foramen as a result of alveolar atrophy. J Oral Rehabil 1995;22(11):831–3.

15. Naitoh M, Hiraiwa Y, Aimiya H, et al. Accessory mental foramen assessment using cone-beam computed tomography. Oral Surg Oral Med Oral Pathol Oral Radiol Endod 2009;107(2):289–94.

16. Jacobs R, Mraiwa N, vanSteenberghe D, et al. Appearance, location, course, and morphology of the mandibular incisive canal: an assessment on spiral CT scan. Dentomaxillofac Radiol 2002;31(5):322–7.

17. Kuribayashi A, Watanabe H, Imaizumi A, et al. Bifid mandibular canals: cone beam computed tomography evaluation. Dentomaxillofac Radiol 2010;39(4):235–9.

18. González-Santana H, Peñarrocha-Diago M, Guarinos-Carbó J, et al. A study of the septa in the maxillary sinuses and the subantral alveolar processes in 30 patients. J Oral Implantol 2007;33(6):340–3.

19. Graves SL. The pterygoid plate implant: a solution for restoring the posterior maxilla. Int J Periodontics Restorative Dent 1994;14(6):512–23.

20. Mardinger O, Namani-Sadan N, Chaushu G, et al. Morphologic changes of the nasopalatine canal related to dental implantation: a radiologic study in different degrees of absorbed maxillae. J Periodontol 2008;79(9):1659–62.

21. Neugebauer J, Ritter L, Mischkowski RA, et al. Evaluation of maxillary sinus anatomy by cone-beam CT prior to sinus floor elevation. Int J Oral Maxillofac Implants 2010;25(2):258–65.

22. Naitoh M, Suenaga Y, Kondo S, et al. Assessment of maxillary sinus septa using cone beam computed tomography: etiological consideration. Clin Implant Dent Relat Res 2009;11(Suppl):e52.

23. Truhlar RS, Orenstein IH, Morris HF, et al. Distribution of bone quality in patients receiving endosseous dental implants. J Oral Maxillofac Surg 1997;55(12 Suppl 5):38–45.

24. Fuh LJ, Huang HL, Chen CS, et al. Variations in bone density at dental implant sites in different regions of the jawbone. J Oral Rehabil 2010;37(5):346–51.

25. Amorfini L, Storelli S, Romeo E. Immediate loading of a fixed complete denture on implants placed with a bone supported surgical computer planned guide: case report. J Oral Implantol 2010;37(Spec No):106–13.

26. Tselios N, Parel SM, Jones JD. Immediate placement and immediate provisional abutment modeling in anterior single-tooth implant restorations using a CAD/CAM application: a clinical report. J Prosthet Dent 2006;95(3):181–5.

27. Turkyilmaz I, Suarez JC, Company AM. Immediate implant placement and provisional crown fabrication after a minimally invasive extraction of a peg-shaped maxillary lateral incisor: a clinical report. J Contemp Dent Pract 2009;10(5):E073–80.

28. Maló P, Rangert B, Nobre M. All-on-4 immediate-function concept with Brånemark System implants for completely edentulous maxillae: a 1-year retrospective clinical study. Clin Implant Dent Relat Res 2005;7(Suppl 1):S88–94.

29. Ostman PO, Hellman M, Sennerby L. Immediate occlusal loading of implants in the partially edentate mandible: a prospective 1-year radiographic and 4-year clinical study. Int J Oral Maxillofac Implants 2008;23(2):315–22.

30. Puig CP. A retrospective study of edentulous patients rehabilitated according to the 'all-on-four' or the 'all-on-six' immediate function concept using flapless computer-guided implant surgery. Eur J Oral Implantol 2010;3(2):155–63.

31. Rocci A, Martignoni M, Gottlow J. Immediate loading in the maxilla using flapless surgery, implants placed in predetermined positions, and prefabricated provisional restorations: a retrospective 3-year clinical study. Clin Implant Dent Relat Res 2003;5(Suppl 1):29–36.

32. Almog DM, Romano PR. CT-based dental imaging for implant planning and surgical guidance. N Y State Dent J 2007;73(1):51–3.

33. Mayer Y, Machtei EE. Divergence correction associated with implant placement: a radiographic study. Int J Oral Maxillofac Implants 2009;24(6):1033–9.

34. Hatcher DC. Operational principles for cone-beam computed tomography. J Am Dent Assoc 2010;141(Suppl 3):3S–6S.

35. Almog DM, Onufrak JM, Hebel K, et al. Comparison between planned prosthetic trajectory and residual bone trajectory using surgical guides and tomography–a pilot study. J Oral Implantol 1995;21(4):275–80.

36. Almog DM, Sanchez R. Correlation between planned prosthetic and residual bone trajectories in dental implants. J Prosthet Dent 1999;81(5):562–7.

37. De Santis D, Canton LC, Cucchi A, et al. Computer-assisted surgery in the lower jaw: double surgical guide for immediately loaded implants in postextractive sites-technical notes and a case report. J Oral Implantol 2010;36(1):61–8.

38. Greenberg AM, Stein JJ. Maxillary sinus grafting and osseointegration surgery. In: Greenberg AM, Prein J, editors. Craniomaxillofacial reconstructive and corrective bone surgery: principles of internal fixation using the AO/ASIF Technique. New York: Springer Verlag; 2002. p. 174–97.

39. Sethi A, Kaus T, Sochor P, et al. Evolution of the concept of angulated abutments in implant dentistry: 14-yearclinical data. Implant Dent 2002;11(1):41–51.

40. Greenberg A. Basics of Cone-Beam CT and CT Guided Dental Implant Surgery. Selected Readings in Oral and Maxillofacial Surgery 2011;19(5):1–48.

Index

Note: Page numbers of article titles are in **boldface** type.

Oral Maxillofacial Surg Clin N Am 27 (2015) 341–344
http://dx.doi.org/10.1016/S1042-3699(15)00021-7
1042-3699/15/$ – see front matter © 2015 Elsevier Inc. All rights reserved.

oralmaxsurgery.theclinics.com

Moving?

Make sure your subscription
moves with you!

To notify us of your new address, find your **Clinics Account Number** (located on your mailing label above your name), and contact customer service at:

Email journalscustomerservice-usa@elsevier.com

800-654-2452 (subscribers in the U.S. & Canada)
314-447-8871 (subscribers outside of the U.S. & Canada)

Fax number: 314-447-8029

Elsevier Health Sciences Division
Subscription Customer Service
3251 Riverport Lane
Maryland Heights, MO 63043

(To ensure uninterrupted delivery of your subscription, please notify us at least 4 weeks in advance of move.)

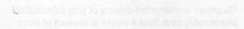

Printed and bound by CPI Group (UK) Ltd, Croydon, CR0 4YY

03/10/2024

01040374-0012